PRAISE FOR

The Barbary Plague

"Irresistible . . . An involving medical detective story, narrated with affection for the period and setting. From Chase's cinematic opening chapter . . . we know we're in expert hands. . . . Richly atmospheric [and] consistently enthralling."   —*The San Francisco Chronicle*

"A pleasure to read, full of people, dramatic situations, individual foibles and collective hard work. I closed the book wishing it had been longer. The story, one hundred years old, has much to teach us about today."   —*The New York Times Book Review*

"Chase, with her elegant, subtle writing, brings alive the human victims, particularly the often-tragic lives of Chinese laborers trying to make a life for themselves."   —*USA Today*

"A story about human nature . . . fear, deceit and denial, and about the handful of purposeful people who managed to overcome these obstacles."   —*The Washington Post*

"A story that highlights the true nature of epidemics—and how employing a combination of acceptance, perseverance and diplomacy are key to solving them . . . The parallels with the AIDS crisis are striking, and the lessons worth salting away for any future epidemics."   —*Publishers Weekly*

"Chase's fast-paced, authoritative account succeeds admirably in capturing the urgency of fighting the plague. No less important is her implicit warning about what happens when politics, greed, and racism become hazardous to the public health."

—*Richmond Times-Dispatch*

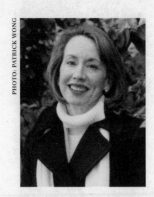

PHOTO: PATRICK WONG

MARILYN CHASE has been a reporter for *The Wall Street Journal* since 1978, concentrating on medical science and health care, and covering stories from cancer and AIDS to bioterrorism; she has been writing about epidemics for the newspaper since 1984. A graduate of Stanford University, Chase was awarded departmental honors in English literature. She attended graduate school at the University of California at Berkeley, earning a master's degree in journalism. Chase lives with her family in San Francisco.

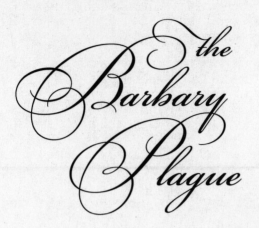

the
Barbary
Plague

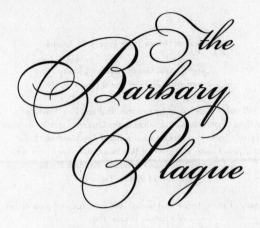

the Barbary Plague

THE BLACK DEATH IN
VICTORIAN SAN FRANCISCO

Marilyn Chase

RANDOM HOUSE TRADE PAPERBACKS / NEW YORK

Grateful acknowledgment is made to the following for permission
to use unpublished material:

DUKE UNIVERSITY RARE BOOK, MANUSCRIPT AND SPECIAL
COLLECTIONS LIBRARY: Selected material from the John Hendricks
Kinyoun Papers housed in the Duke University Rare Book,
Manuscript and Special Collections Library.
COLBY BUXTON RUCKER: Images of W. Colby Rucker as well as
quotes from his diary, autobiography, and other papers. Material
used courtesy of Colby Buxton Rucker.

Library of Congress Cataloging-in-Publication Data
Chase, Marilyn
The Barbary plague: the black death in Victorian San
Francisco/Marilyn Chase.
p. cm.
ISBN 0-375-75708-2
1. Plague—California—San Francisco—History—20th century.
I. Title.
RC176.C2 C48 2003   362.1'969232'0979461—dc21   2002068102

Random House website address: www.atrandom.com
Printed in the United States of America
2 4 6 8 9 7 5 3 1

Book design by Judith Stagnitto Abbate

For Randy, Jack, and Becca

Contents

Downtown San Francisco at the Turn of the Century

N

San Francisco Bay

Fort Mason

LOBOS SQUARE

Columbus Ave.
(Montgomery Ave.)

LATIN QUARTER

WASHINGTON SQUARE

Union St.

CHINATOWN

Ferry Building

Broadway

Old Globe Hotel

PORTSMOUTH SQUARE

Pacific St.

Spofford Alley

Merchant St.

Jackson St.

Waverly Place

U.S. Marine Hospital Service
Morgue and Laboratory

Washington St.

ALTA PLAZA

Lafayette Park

Clay St.

Sacramento St.

California St.

Powell St.

Stockton St.

Dupont St.

Kearny St.

Pine St.

Bush St.

Sutter St.

UNION SQUARE

Palace Hotel

Post St.

Geary St.

SOUTH OF MARKET

Filmore St.

HAMILTON SQUARE

Market St.

JEFFERSON SQUARE

Polk St.

Van Ness Ave.

Mission St.

CIVIC CENTER/
CITY HALL

ALAMO SQUARE

"The Rattery"

Page St.

Market St.

MISSION DISTRICT

City and County Hospital

MARIN COUNTY

San Francisco Bay

Tiburon

Angel Island

Alcatraz

Yerba Buena Island

Pacific Ocean

SAN FRANCISCO

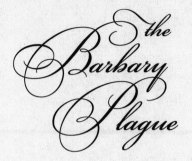

the Barbary Plague

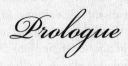

Prologue

SAN FRANCISCO IN 1900 was a Gold Rush boomtown settling into a gaudy middle age. Fifty years earlier, it had been a miners' camp pitched upon sand dunes. Now it had a pompous new skyline with skyscrapers nearly twenty stories tall, grand hotels, and Victorian mansions on Nob Hill. Cable cars scaled its hills on chains that jingled like the necklace on a vaudeville soubrette. The city filled three opera houses with the zeal of the nouveaux riches. But underneath its ermine opera cape beat the heart of its rowdy past: the old Barbary Coast was still alive in the saloons and vaudevilles, bawdy houses and "French restaurants," with dining downstairs and women upstairs.

Keening seagulls rode the cool currents of fog and sun, circling town with their rusty cries. At street level, the city (while eager to embrace electricity and motorcars) still lived on gaslight and horsepower. Horse-drawn buggies and streetcars rattled west from downtown, past churches, temples, and sandlots, toward Ocean Beach. The oblique slash of Market Street bisected the town, running from southwest to northeast, from Castro Street, past the dome of City Hall, past the Palace Hotel, past the Emporium and Golden Rule Bazaar department store, and finally ending at the water's edge, where the Ferry Building's clock tower was a traveler's first view of the city.

The wharf bristled with masts and smokestacks from as many as a thousand sailing ships and steamers arriving each year. To guide their passage through the fog, lighthouses pulsed from every promontory.

Decades before modern foghorns, each island in the bay—Angel Island, Alcatraz, and Yerba Buena—had its own sound signature from fog bells, ship's whistles, sirens, or chimes. On foggy days, the bay must have sounded like an antique calliope, playing its strange music to guide ships' captains through corridors of mist to a safe harbor.[1]

But the harbor would not be safe for long. Across the Pacific came an unexpected import, bubonic plague. Sailing from China and Hawaii into the unbridged arms of the Golden Gate, it arrived aboard vessels bearing rich cargoes, hopeful immigrants, and infected vermin. The rats slipped out of their shadowy holds, scuttled down the rigging, and alighted on the wharf. Uphill they scurried, insinuating themselves into the heart of the city.

Two doctors in federal uniform—Joseph Kinyoun and Rupert Blue—would each try in his own way to quell the pestilence. One doctor would try to subdue the outbreak from his laboratory at the quarantine station on Angel Island. The other doctor would work at street level, purging the infection from boardwalk to basement. The public health efforts of the day were handicapped by limited scientific knowledge and bedeviled by the twin demons of denial and discrimination. One man would fail, and the other would succeed to become the top physician in the land. Today, few people know their names. But their mission would foreshadow the challenges posed by epidemics for the century to come.

When plague hit, one doctor would later recall, "We were fighting in the dark." The scientists were an unwelcome presence in the city by the Golden Gate. Turn-of-the-century San Francisco aspired to be not a plague zone, but the "Paris of the Pacific." Its mayor, James Phelan, a proponent of the "City Beautiful" movement, sought to build its civic center into a Beaux Arts showplace. In industry, the city was proud to be the shipping power of the Pacific Coast and the western transit center for the U.S. military. As evidenced by the city's motto, "Gold in peace, iron in war," San Francisco's fortunes were forged to metal, bright or dull. Its tycoons got rich by mining ore from the hills and building great banking houses in its financial district. Later, ironworks and shipbuilders kept the city afloat by supplying warships for the Spanish-American War in the Philippines.[2]

The Spirit of 1900, in a *Chronicle* newspaper artist's rendering, depicted the goddess of progress operating a railroad, a telegraph, and a dynamo engine. San Franciscans embraced this ethic of progress, damming the Hetch Hetchy River and razing the Tahoe forest for power and building material—and drawing protests from the aging John Muir and his infant Sierra Club. From boardrooms to church pulpits, the city cheered the Spanish-American conflict as a boon to its economy. As the Union Iron Works and the Southern Pacific Railroad went, so went the city. Sons of the Gold Rush, San Franciscans styled themselves as a new breed of Argonauts, explorers and executors of manifest destiny.[3]

If the East had the Astors, Carnegies, and Mellons, San Francisco had the "Big Four" railroad barons—Hopkins, Huntington, Crocker, and Stanford—who clustered their palazzi on Nob Hill like Renaissance princes occupying a Tuscan hill town. Soon, other industrialists followed them, abandoning the south of Market Street for the fresher climes of Nob Hill and Pacific Heights, where their mansions mushroomed in a hodgepodge of architectural styles—Italian Renaissance, French baroque, Victorian, Edwardian, and Queen Anne—all elbowing one another for supremacy.

On sunny weekends, a caravan of horse buggies, landaus, calèches, and a few rattletrap automobiles faced into the wind, rambling west through Golden Gate Park, whose green carpet replaced the sand dunes and tamed the sandstorms that once scoured the city's western fringes. Gliding through the canopy of manicured greenery, the day-trippers rolled on to the gingerbread castle of Cliff House, a wooden Victorian restaurant perched on a promontory overlooking the breakers of the Pacific Ocean and barking sea lions on Seal Rock. Their destination reached, the caravan turned and rolled home, merry and windburned, ahead of the fog that blew in from the west. The weekly parade lasted all day.[4]

Strollers ambled on Market, Montgomery, or Kearny Street. Men wore broad-shouldered tweeds and bowlers. Ladies, corseted into breathless figure eights, swept past in day gowns of ecru, coral, and celestial blue from fine stores like the White House or the City of Paris. Picture hats resembling platters of meringue and Tuscan straw bonnets were all the rage, crowned with sprays of heliotrope, bunches of cherries, or egret feathers in a nest of net. Sailor-suited children, sated with peanuts and French caramels, trailed their parents home from the matinee.[5]

At home, supper waited. In those days, Kona coffee cost 20 cents a pound, ocean fish went for 12½ cents a pound, California figs were four pounds for a quarter. Sourdough bread, the Gold Rush staple, cost a dime for two loaves.

Theaters were packed, and there was a spectacle for every taste, from a staging of Mark Twain's *Pudd'nhead Wilson* to a piano recital by Paderewski. There was a French farce at the Alcazar Theatre. The dashing maestro Walter Damrosch conducted *The Flying Dutchman* at the opera house. Golden youth of the upper classes waltzed demurely at the Greenway balls and the La Jeunesse Cotillions. Showgirls and young swells danced the "buck and wing."

Once the tycoons migrated to Nob Hill, the working class took over the sunny triangle south of Market Street, turning it from a fashionable neighborhood into a utilitarian zone of boardinghouses and flats. There, a good time was the penny vaudeville or, better yet, free amateur night at Kapp & Street's Tamale Grotto and Refined Concert Hall, a Market Street establishment that advertised itself as "A Strictly First-Class Vaudeville Show." In some ways, the town itself was a vaudeville show. But those abandoned by the boomtown often ended their misery with a searing gulp of carbolic acid or an open gaslight jet with the keyhole stuffed tight. For those who survived their misfortune, the last resort was the almshouse on the foggy, windward side of Twin Peaks.

Newcomers to the port of San Francisco sailed or steamed through the Golden Gate and waited while their vessel lay at anchor in the bay's quarantine station off Angel Island. If you were Chinese, they probed your glands, peered into your throat, and bathed you with disinfectants. If you were white, the doctors spared you the antiseptic baptism. However, you still had to open your mouth for the doctors, and your luggage for the inspectors, before landing at the dock of the Pacific Mail Steamship Company.

The long, low, shedlike warehouse maintained separate reception rooms for the arrival of whites and Chinese. In one room, Victorian travelers disembarked and reunited with their families after a Hawaiian cruise. In another room, immigrants in their padded jackets and cloth shoes were received. Women in silken coats and tiny platformed sandals were claimed by their husbands. Fresh-cheeked country girls were delivered over to madams who dressed in black and wore rings of keys to their cribs in the flesh trade.[6]

Wagons carried them uphill to Chinatown. A dozen blocks in the heart of the city, Chinatown was a village of balconied brick-and-wooden tenements, incense-spiced temples, groceries hung with mahogany-glazed ducks, pyramids of onions and cabbage, and mounds of oranges and pale jade melons.

Sheltering as many as twenty thousand to thirty thousand Chinese, the neighborhood was a teeming outpost of the empire of China transplanted to the Barbary Coast. To the observer, it was visibly a bachelor society, a colony of mostly male laborers sporting American bowler hats atop their traditional queues. Most lived lean, solitary lives in rooming houses, for it was costly to bring families to San Francisco. Wives and children—usually those of wealthy merchants—were in the minority. Barred from attending school with whites, Chinese children were consigned to a segregated school that stopped at the sixth grade.

Whether denizens or California-born, Chinatown's people relied on the powerful merchants of the Chinese Six Companies to speak for them. It was a consortium of district associations, composed of people who had come from various regions of China. Also known as the Chinese Benevolent Association, the group wore many hats: It was part philanthropic society, part informal diplomatic corps, and part Chamber of Commerce. It raised funds for the poor, fought bias, and mediated between Chinatown and the city's white power structure. When turf wars broke out between the tongs—secret societies that controlled gambling and prostitution—the Chinese Six Companies played peacemaker. When Caucasian law discriminated against the Chinese, the Six Companies hired lawyers and went to court. A council of elders for the expatriate community, it helped its people navigate a turbulent white society while they lived, and return their bones to China when they died.

Chinatown's main thoroughfare was Dupont Street, *Do bahn gai* in the local dialect. City fathers would later rename it Grant Avenue, but it remains Dupont Street among the old-timers to this day. To the west rose the hotels and mansions of Nob Hill. To the east stretched the financial district, the dockside shipping companies, and the gray silken mirror of the bay. To the south lay the smart shops, restaurants, and theaters—as well as the brothels—clustered near Union Square. To the north were the Barbary Coast saloons and the Latin Quarter, where Romance languages filled the air and bohemian artists met over rough red wine. Few of these enticements were open to Asians—especially poor Asian laborers.[7]

Victorian men in bowlers and women in prim shirtwaists came to Chinatown to gawk. Some sipped tea and bought curios. For a few coins, others hired a guide to lead them on a tour through the opium dens. They could watch as the smokers reclined on narrow bunks, cradling the paraphernalia of their bliss in a horn box. First they melted the tarry ball of poppy sap on a wire, and then they packed the bubbling, viscous paste into thimble-size stone pipes fitted with long, thin bamboo stems. Then they sipped the pungent fumes, refilling their pipes again and again, until they reached Xanadu, going slack and glassy-eyed at the vision. Some tourists recoiled at the sickly scent of burning poppy sap, while others likened it to roasting peanuts. There were other secret parlors, the guides confided, off-limits to tourists, where even white men and women partook of the pipe.[8]

Of course, Chinatown had no monopoly on vice. It's said the storyteller Jack London and his friends democratically surveyed cribs of every color.[9] Indeed, the epicenter of downtown vice was Morton Street, an alley just off Union Square, where the women were boldly displayed in the shop windows. Later the city would rechristen the passage Maiden Lane.

Chinatown was born, just as greater San Francisco had been, when the glint of gold drew the eyes of fortune seekers. During the 1850s, thousands of men fled their rural villages in the Pearl River Delta of Guangdong Province, whose capital city is Canton, or Guangzhou. They spent weeks at sea in a dark and vile steerage in order to reach the land they called Gamsaan—"Gold Mountain." In the 1860s, the railroad bosses recruited still more Chinese to help them blast through the Sierras, lay the track, and pound the spikes of the transcontinental railroad. When those jobs were done, the Chinese left the mines and the rails to pick plums and cut asparagus, following the harvest seasons from the fields of California to as far north as the orchards of Washington and the fisheries of Alaska.

In town, the Chinese washed clothes, stitched shirts, cobbled shoes, and rolled cigars. At the Palace Hotel, they worked as cooks or donned livery as doormen, wielding scoops after the horses that clopped into the carriage entrance. They were butlers and chefs for the hostesses of the haut monde. As laborers, they were discreet, hardworking, and cheap. As small-business owners, they helped form a rising merchant class. Their industry was rewarded with plenty of work in the land of the Stars and Stripes, or, as they called America, "the flowery flag nation." They became indispensable.

As long as times were good, the Chinese were accepted, but a late-nineteenth-century depression turned the tide. Formerly prized for their productivity, the Chinese now were cast as cunning and insidious job stealers. The incendiary white labor leader Dennis Kearney stirred up sandlot rallies that turned into riots under the war cry "The Chinese must go."[10] Cobblers in the White Labor League stamped their shoes with a mark that guaranteed that no Chinese hand had worked the leather. By buying Caucasian products, consumers were told, "[y]ou will be helping the White shoemakers of this city and State to support themselves and their families."[11] Soon the scapegoating broadened. Chinese were blamed not only for stealing work from white men, but for corrupting the city's youth with opium and prostitution and for spreading disease.[12]

Politicians moved to mollify these fears through passage of the Chinese Exclusion Act in 1882, a law barring the entry of so-called coolie labor. The very word *coolie*—from the Indian *Kulī*—conjures up low-caste laborers or bearers of burdens for white masters. As the twentieth century dawned, colonial condescension still engendered hostility that often boiled over into acts of violence.

Strolling the boardwalks and cobblestone streets of San Francisco in 1900, one might see a Chinese man get his queue yanked hard or even chopped off. The long, jet pigtail was a sign of loyalty to the Manchu Dynasty, and a passport home if things became unbearable. Some say these clashes between East and West gave birth to the word *hoodlum*—after the cry of "Huddle 'em!" shouted by young white toughs accosting a Chinese victim. This might seem fanciful, but even if apocryphal, it holds a kernel of truth.[13]

On Sunday near the First Congregational Church, one might see what the writer Ambrose Bierce once witnessed: a gang of Sunday schoolers stoning a Chinese man walking on Dupont Street, until the processional hymn called them in to prayer.[14]

A Chinese laundryman who went into a white saloon to play dice was stuffed into his laundry basket, thrown outside, and robbed to buy drinks for the house. When he went to court seeking justice, a lawyer and judge mocked him. The newspapers portrayed the case as low comedy and the assault as a good-natured attempt to "subdue the Chink's luck and sporty ways."[15]

San Francisco papers pandered openly to the fears of white workers, with "Chink" cartoons depicting caricatured immigrants spouting pidgin. In popular parlance, they were "the heathen Chinee"—a phrase coined by Bret Harte in his verse "Plain Language from Truthful James," telling of a wily gambler, Ah Sin, who hides cards up his sleeve and cheats white men out of their pay.[16] Amid rising paranoia over the "yellow peril," the caricature of the bland but cunning outsider burned its way into the psyche of Victorian San Francisco. Just as the economic depression had strangled tolerance, so disease outbreaks further fanned race resentments. Poised on the threshold of the Pacific Rim, San Francisco had always been open to imported disease. Now, in 1900, it was about to receive the most famous scourge in history.

Bubonic plague had ravaged Europe, from fourteenth-century Florence to seventeenth-century London. It smoldered along the Himalayan borderlands between India and China into the late nineteenth century. As soldiers crisscrossed the borders, they brought plague into China's interior, where it flared to a ferocious epidemic that erupted in Hong Kong in 1894. From that port, plague embarked aboard ships sailing to many continents. Among its destinations was the city by the Golden Gate.

Plague traveled in stealth. No one yet knew how it spread. Nineteenth-century theories of its transmission focused on dirt, tainted food, and a "miasma," or cloud of infectious vapors. In the boomtown of San Francisco, the business and political elite believed plague to be an alien scourge that would tarnish their trade and tourism. So from City Hall to the dome of the state capitol, officials dismissed the threat. The little people would die of it while the powerful debated its existence.

In 1900, the city played an active role in courting catastrophe. Like most Victorian cities, San Francisco neglected its aging sewer system, fouled its bay with garbage, and tolerated a burgeoning population of rats. Victorian cities were a petri dish for all manner of epidemics—like diphtheria, tuberculosis, and smallpox—and none more so than San Francisco. Whispers of "pesthouse" sent a stab of fear through families who never knew when their neighbors would be bundled into an ambulance buggy and carted off to an isolation ward of the county hospital. Mysterious germs, which no one but scientists could see, ran rampant until they closed throats with a white membrane, eroded lungs with coughing, or embossed faces with scars.[17]

With almost a tenth of the city terraced into its twelve tiny blocks, Chinatown was especially vulnerable to disease. But sickness on Dupont Street, unlike sickness elsewhere, was viewed by city officials as a symptom of alien squalor. Whites held their noses at Chinatown's smoky stew of scents, as if the very air were a cloud of contagion. Even in medical circles, some doctors cleaved to old notions that the poor and sick could infect others through their exhalations. Another local myth held that Chinatown's haze—mingling temple incense, pork smokehouses, and opium vapors—was noxious to white nostrils but rendered the denizens immune to the diseases they bred. The Chinese were blamed for the crowding and dilapidation of Chinatown, even though bias barred them from living elsewhere.

For the record, City Hall had published its view of Chinatown's health a generation earlier, in an 1885 report to the San Francisco Board of Supervisors:

> The Chinese brought here with them and successfully maintained and perpetuated the grossest habits of bestiality practiced by the human race [gambling, opium, and prostitution]. . . . [They] have innoculated our youth not only with the virus of immorality in its most hideous form, but have through the same sources physically poisoned the blood of thousands by the innoculation with diseases the most frightful that the flesh is heir to, and furnishing posterity with a line of scrofulous and leprous victims that might better never have been born than to curse themselves and mankind at large with their contagious presence.[18]

Against this backdrop of blame, the new threat arrived. At first, it was only dimly perceived. Dispatches from Hong Kong told of a violent outbreak, harrowing people living a continent away. But by 1899, steamers and sailing ships were carrying the infection across the Pacific to Hawaii. Cases of fever and swollen glands, followed by a swift death, occurred in Honolulu's Chinatown. Recognizing that plague had arrived, the city's health department ordered that the plague houses be burned. But a freak twist of trade winds whipped the flames out of control, igniting a church steeple and throwing a fountain of sparks beyond the reach of fire hoses. Soon Chinatown was engulfed, the flames touching off explosions in fireworks sheds and reducing shops to ashes. When the smoke cleared, six thousand Chinese were homeless in Honolulu.[19]

Learning the fate of their countrymen in the islands, San Francisco's Chinese were terror-stricken. It seemed a double curse: epidemic followed by fire. But white San Franciscans felt tropical pestilence could never trouble their hometown, with its cool and misty climate. Capturing this naive optimism, the *San Francisco Examiner* ran a story headlined WHY SAN FRANCISCO IS PLAGUE-PROOF.[20]

Safe inside their red velvet drawing rooms with brocaded curtains and satin-covered spittoons, powerful San Franciscans were certain that this Asian plague could never gain a foothold in a city that had bel canto and porcelain bathtubs. The specter of plague was like a wraith in the fog, impossible to grasp.

But plague scares had seized the city before. A year earlier, the Japanese vessel *Nippon Maru* reached the city after a Pacific crossing marred by two plague deaths. On entering San Francisco Bay, two Asian stowaways jumped overboard. Their bodies were fished from the cold gray swells, still wearing *Nippon Maru* life preservers. Doctors who performed an autopsy found suspicious-looking germs.[21]

But isolating the cause of death is difficult in a decomposing corpse, where all manner of bacteria run wild. Experts disputed the stowaways' cause of death. And the fate of the *Nippon Maru*—with two dead at sea and two dead in port—was soon forgotten.

On the eve of 1900, another ship appeared on the horizon: the four-masted steamship *Australia,* making her regular run from Hawaii to the Golden Gate. Around Christmas 1899, when San Franciscans were trimming their trees, the ship had lain at anchor in the infected port of Honolulu. Then the *Australia* took on cargo, weighed anchor, and made way for San Francisco.

On New Year's Day 1900, the San Francisco newspapers noted the imminent arrival of the *Australia*. Stiff southwesterly winds chased the rain and scoured the skies. On January 2 she appeared, as long as a football field, knifing through the steel blue water and into the Golden Gate. She anchored at the quarantine station off Angel Island, while officers searched her from stateroom to steerage. They failed to find any traces of infection, and under constant pressure from impatient shippers, the quarantine officers had no choice but to grant her permission to land.

So the *Australia*'s bladelike hull turned away from Angel Island toward the port of San Francisco. With a touch of unease, the quarantine officers watched as the V-shaped spume widened in her wake. Easing into the dock, the *Australia* delivered the sanitized bags of her sixty-eight passengers and a shipment of fumigated mail, along with some four-legged stowaways that, somehow, escaped detection.[22]

The Year of the Rat

◈

THE NEW YEAR OF 1900 ushered in dangerous times. In San Francisco, it was, as always, a holiday with two faces. Downtown, white celebrants raised their usual end-of-year ruckus. In the streets of Chinatown, a shadow fell over the Lunar New Year, in an ominous prologue to the year ahead.

Rain spattered the boardwalks on New Year's Eve. When the skies cleared, the merrymakers came out. A band of maskers gathered on the corner of Market and Kearny streets, just below Union Square and Chinatown. Blowing horns and clanging cowbells, they hurled confetti and thrashed passersby with evergreen boughs left over from Christmas. Then the celebration turned ugly. Charging north up Kearny for five blocks, the carousers reached Chinatown and started grabbing Chinese musical instruments from the shops, banging the gongs, and blasting away on the winds. The din was so loud, it pierced the paneled recesses of the nearby men's clubs. Bystanders cringed to hear the strains of "Auld Lang Syne" mingling with what sounded like the minor wails of a Chinese funeral band.[1]

But funereal sentiments were very much in order in the year 1900. For death was the uninvited guest at this New Year's feast although, like the maskers, it came in disguise.

In Chinatown, the approach of the Chinese New Year—the turning over of the lunar calendar in February—usually was heralded by the hiss and bang of firecrackers, warding off demons and trailing smoke that pricked the nostrils with excitement. Sidewalk stands traditionally sold stacks of juicy sugarcane and mounds of crackling melon seeds. To perfume the spring banquet tables, people would buy pots of narcissus bulbs, crowned with stiff green shoots and buds that burst into white trumpets with a center of gold that symbolized good fortune. People wearing silk tunics in peacock hues would call on family and friends with gifts and cakes. Children in embroidered skullcaps and jeweled headdresses would parade hand in hand.

All this would happen in a festive Lunar New Year. But not in this year of 1900. Instead of fireworks, gunfire rang through the streets, and the alleys ran with blood. Gang warfare had struck again. As punishment, the San Francisco Police Department cracked down on the whole district, canceling all holiday celebrations. Sidewalks were barren of flowers, parties were banned, and the streets were still.

So the Chinese New Year crept in, as gray and drab as its namesake on the great wheel of the astrological calendar, for 1900 was the Year of the Rat.

According to Chinese astrology, people born in the Year of the Rat are clever and resourceful. Family loving to the point of being clannish, rats are also frugal, sharp-witted, and good companions in adversity.[2]

This year, however, rats were to become harbingers of evil. Merchants awoke to find grizzled pelts of dead vermin in their alleyways and courtyards. Dull-eyed, stiff, shaggy cadavers sent a shudder through the neighborhood.

In the old country, they portended epidemics—in any house where rats had died, human deaths were sure to follow. In 1792, the poet Shih Tao-Nan had written:

> *The coming of the devil of plague*
> *Suddenly makes the lamp dim,*
> *Then it is blown out,*
> *Leaving man, ghost and corpse in the dark room.*[3]

In the old country, households would flee at the sight of a dead rodent. But here, there was nowhere else to go. Discrimination hindered Chinese from living elsewhere in town. Fearing an avalanche of bad luck in the New Year, they filed complaints with the city. As usual, nothing was done. Many people considered rats as the inevitable companions of human settlements, even as natural garbage collectors performing a salutary service. And this was, after all, Chinatown.

March blew in, raw and unsettled. In the late winter mist, a fever stole up from the waterfront. It skulked in on four legs, and invaded the bunks of the working poor who slept layered in dense tenements.

Many kinds of illness, from typhoid to diphtheria, raked the city's poor. But this disease was different. This was the scourge that for centuries had come in the wake of a rat invasion. When the rats died, the fleas abandoned their corpses, seeking new blood, human blood, in the warrens of the poor. The disease attacked with a violent rush of fever and shuddering chills. A headache seemed to core out the skull. Victims weakened and took to their beds. Penetrating pains raked the back and limbs. Red lumps erupted from the armpits and groin, excruciating to the touch. Hemorrhages would burst beneath the skin, causing black bruises. Senses wandering, the sick would chatter and fidget restlessly, plucking at their bedclothes. Their agitation subsided only as they sank into a coma, ending in death.

Late on the afternoon of Tuesday, March 6, 1900, the phone rang at the police headquarters. A dead man was in the Chinese undertaker's shop at 814 Clay Street, and the police physician needed to issue a burial certificate. The corpse bore no gross signs of foul play, no bulletholes or knife wounds, but the man had died of a violent disease.

The dead man's name was Wong Chut King. He was a forty-one-year-old lumber salesman, living the lean life of a bachelor laborer in the Globe Hotel at 1001 Dupont Street on the corner of Jackson. The Globe Hotel, a once fashionable spot turned flophouse, was known as the "Five Stories." Its cramped cells sheltered hundreds of Chinatown's workingmen, sharing their life of expansive dreams and narrow bunks in their adopted land.

Now he was middle-aged and sick. When he felt too weak to drag himself to work at the lumberyard, Wong Chut King took to his spartan quarters at the Globe. The gaslight shed a weak gold halo over the bunk where Wong lay, drawing his knees up to cradle a knot of pain that pulsed in his groin. He shifted uneasily on his cot. Local healers offered herbs to ease his aches, ascribed to a cranky middle-aged bladder. A fierce fever made him sweat and shiver by turns. He threw up his last meager meal. He fell into a fiery delirium.

As his fever soared, his mind became unmoored, floating freely in and out of consciousness. Where Wong wandered in his delirium—back to his native village or on to some fever dream of Gold Mountain—only he could see. Perhaps in febrile visions, Wong saw his barren cell pulse with unearthly colors. Perhaps he saw himself as a young man, leaving his village of Pei Hang, in the county of Ling Yup.[4] Crossing the Pacific to Gold Mountain, he discovered a town more gray than gold. Perhaps he saw himself in the sea of Chinatown bachelors, growing old an ocean away from their families, easing their bones by visiting "hundred-men's-wives" in brothels called "green mansions."[5]

Now, as Wong sank, the bacteria flourished in his glands and blood. Although it takes few plague bacteria to cause infection, the flea that bit Wong probably injected a lethal dose of fifteen thousand bacteria. Like most victims, he likely would have scratched at the bite, driving the germs deeper. At once they multiplied, spreading from the flea bite on his leg up toward the lymph node in his pelvis. Lymph glands, the sentries of the immune system, struggled to contain the invaders. The lymph node grew swollen, inflamed, and tender to the touch. His fever rose. His tongue turned white and furry, and sores crusted his lips. Eventually the infection spilled over into his bloodstream. Giant germ-eating cells—macrophages—rushed to devour the plague bacteria but were overcome. Some bacteria were killed by antibodies that converged on the scene. But as they died, the bacteria detonated a final weapon—deadly toxins. These poisons ran riot in the blood, vandalizing the tissues of the heart, liver, and spleen. Under this assault, the organs began to hemorrhage and disintegrate. Vessels dilated, and blood pressure plunged. Septic shock set in. Wong Chut King descended into a coma.[6]

Bad luck was believed to visit any house where a tenant died, so Wong's inert body was hauled from the Globe's basement and carried to a nearby coffin shop. The *sau pan po* was literally a shop for selling "long-life boards."[7] But there, Wong's life ended. His agonal gasps slowed, their intervals lengthening. His chest contracted. He exhaled his last breath.

When police surgeon F. P. Wilson arrived at the Wing Sang coffin shop, he unwrapped the corpse. His fingers began palpating the contours of Wong's livid form, where rigor mortis was beginning to set in. His fingers found the swollen lymph glands. Plainly visible on the dead man's thigh was a small sore, festering where Wong had scratched at some irritation. Perhaps it was an insect bite. The police surgeon sent for city health officer A. P. O'Brien. Together they telephoned a young city bacteriologist named Wilfred Kellogg.

As midnight approached, Wilson, O'Brien, and Kellogg performed a postmortem examination, mining the body for clues. They pierced the lumps and withdrew fluid from the knot of inflamed glands. They extracted blood and straw-colored lymph fluid, with bits of pink pulpy tissue from the body, saving it for analysis. Under the microscope lens, a swarm of bacteria swam into focus—clusters of short, rod-shaped germs with rounded tips that, when stained, turned pink and looked like closed safety pins.

It looked suspiciously like plague.

Plague reports had been trickling out of Hong Kong and Hawaii for some time, putting the city's health officers on alert for any sudden death from fever. But the city's bacteriology laboratory needed to confirm these suspicions. A final diagnosis required a senior expert, someone with a more sophisticated lab outfit and time to corroborate the findings. They knew where to find such an expert, at the quarantine station on Angel Island, but city officials didn't wait for a definitive diagnosis.

Police officers descended on Chinatown in the darkness, stringing ropes around its dozen square blocks. Whites were ushered out of Chinatown, and the Chinese were sealed inside. Panic exploded among the confined. Some raced the length of the barriers, pacing the perimeter, looking for a way out. But police patrolled the barricades, clubs at the ready. Only police and health officers could cross the cordon sanitaire.

Making his evening rounds, a reporter for *Chung Sai Yat Po,* the Chinatown daily newspaper, saw the siege unfold. He raced back to the newspaper headquarters to prepare his report:

> The Caucasian doctor examining the body was shocked to find that the person died of an epidemic illness. That is why they put the quarantine on Chinatown to prevent spreading

of the disease. Alas, the epidemic was caused by the imbal-
ance of Qi, the energy of the four seasons. It cannot be spread
from person to person. . . . By Friday, it is hoped that we will
know that this was not the plague. Otherwise what happened
in Honolulu might happen to us.[8]

"Honolulu"—fear clutched the throats of all who whispered the
word. Chinatown's residents knew all about the incineration of Honolulu just a couple of months earlier. As the crowds milled about in
increasing alarm, they watched as Wong Chut King's clothes and bedding were pitched into the street and set alight. Flames crackled and
smoke curled up, showering ashes like gray snow. Health officers
lugged in sulfur pots and began fumigating the coffin shop. The air
smelled of rotten eggs. Wong's body was wrapped in a linen shroud
that had been soaked in an antiseptic solution of bichloride of mercury and sealed in a lead coffin lined with powdery chloride of lime.
The coffin was loaded onto a horse cart and driven over cobblestones
west of downtown to the Odd Fellows Cemetery. There, the body was
given to the flames.

Autopsy and cremation was the fate prescribed by health departments for any victim of an epidemic disease. But cutting and burning
of the body violated the Confucian principle of filial piety. Autopsy
was considered an affront to the parents of the deceased, who gave
him life; and cremation was the final desecration. Such practices left
a disembodied spirit in the void. "The ashes will be scattered in the
air," wrote the reporter for the Chinese daily, "and let go to the home
of nothingness, the cave of emptiness."[9]

Chinatown had its own view of what ailed Wong Chut King, and
it was certainly not the plague. Elders confided that the lumberman,
like many bachelor workers who visited the green mansions—suffered
from "notorious gonorrhea," also known as "poisonous mango-shaped
lump."[10]

In a community of lonely laborers living a continent away from
their wives, such ills were as common an occupational hazard as callused hands. Although venereal disease was an unsavory topic, it
would not bring down the fiery retribution on the neighborhood that
was promised by a diagnosis of plague.

Speculation about the torching of the Globe Hotel reached the ears of its tenants, who fled their bunks and vanished like smoke. But the Globe wasn't burned to the ground. Instead, the city continued its chemical assault, fumigating and spraying acrid chemicals in hopes of purging the disease. The sanitation had its drawbacks. The smoking pots of sulfur smudged paint, spoiled hangings, and ruined upholstery. In neighboring stores, it would yellow pale silks and silt carvings with gritty smoke residue. Thick, rank clouds blinded residents with tears and sent them choking and sputtering into the streets for air. If the disease didn't kill them, they guessed the cure surely would.

The confined stared longingly at the world outside the cordon. Outside were jobs, money, food. A brave and foolhardy few tried to vault over or slip under the barricades. The crack of a billy club brought the escapees back into quarantine.

From his official residence in Chinatown, the Chinese consul, Ho Yow, watched the street scene unfold below with a leaden heart.

At home in two worlds, Ho spoke perfect English but posed for portraits in the traditional silk robes and dark silk skullcap of a senior Asian diplomat. Although he was his country's designated representative of Chinese culture, he enjoyed Western sports like harness racing, and he raced his champion mare, Solo, all over Northern California. Solo trotted to victory behind a driver clad in red-and-blue racing silks, embroidered with a magnificent dragon with shimmering scales and flashing eyes.

Ho knew well the danger of Black Death. In his father's household in China, two servants had died of plague.[11] But, he argued, blockading the whole district was discrimination. Anyone could see the quarantine rope markedly zigzagged to exclude white stores on the boundaries of Chinatown.

More than the plague itself, Consul Ho feared that the quarantine would provoke a relapse of exclusion-law fever. He begged the city to be fair to his people. Immigrants born in China were barred from becoming naturalized U.S. citizens. They were legally subjects of the emperor of China. Even Chinese people born in America hadn't been deemed citizens until two years earlier, when the 1898 U.S. Supreme Court formally recognized their status in the case of Wong Kim Ark. Still, in the eyes of the white majority, their Asian features and golden hue stamped them indelibly as aliens.

Ho sought out the Chinese Six Companies. More than just a Chinese Chamber of Commerce, the group functioned as de facto diplomats, working with the consul to keep peace between the tongs and untangle immigration snarls. Now, facing quarantine, Ho and the Chinese Six Companies had another mission: protecting the civil rights of their people. So they hired lawyers and vowed to defend their small stake in America.

On Gold Mountain in the Year of the Rat, the bad times were about to get worse.

"A Lively Corpse"

◉

CRADLING AUTOPSY SAMPLES from Wong Chut King in glass vials, city bacteriologist Wilfred Kellogg boarded a streetcar. When the driver signaled the Ferry Building stop, Kellogg got off and bought a ticket for Angel Island. Ascending the ramp to board the ferry, he no doubt saw the water afloat with garbage, the screaming gulls swooping down to pluck tidbits from the waves, and the rats gorging at low tide.

The ferry churned north, over waters ruffled into whitecaps by the stiff bay winds. Past the stony outcrop of Alcatraz, the ferry continued on toward to the tree-dotted, tan hulk of Angel Island. In mid-bay, as the ferry slapped over swells, Kellogg clutched his samples more tightly for safety. One misstep could send the stoppered tubes crashing to the cabin floor, and the translucent pink lymph fluid and bits of bloody pulp would be lost amid shards of glass. The mystery of Wong's death would remain unsolved.

Forty minutes later, the vessel swung around the north side of Angel Island, cut its engines, and nosed into Hospital Cove. Kellogg steadied his sea legs and lurched down the ramp onto the pier, then walked on to the headquarters of the quarantine officer, Joseph J. Kinyoun. Kinyoun's job was to inspect arriving ships, check the passengers and crew, isolate the sick, fumigate the cargo, and keep diseases out of the country. It was his duty to impose federal standards of hygiene on this port city that, after Washington, D.C., must have seemed like a frontier outpost. Sent to San Francisco from the capital just ten months before, he was a disease warrior. Angel Island was his fortress, and all San Francisco Bay was his moat.

Kinyoun was a "Pasteurian," a doctor trained in Europe in the new science of bacteriology founded by the patriarch of infectious diseases, Louis Pasteur. He was thirty-nine years old, portly and balding, with a cleft chin and an obstinate streak. He had a tender ego and a gut to match. Kinyoun was unsuited to his politically turbulent job. A public health officer needs the hide of a pachyderm, he told colleagues.[1] Instead, he had the skin of an onion.

Conceived on the eve of the Civil War, Joseph James Kinyoun was born in East Bend, North Carolina, in November 1860. The son of a Confederate army surgeon, John Hendricks Kinyoun, and his wife, Bettie Ann, Kinyoun spent his infancy in the care of his mother, who prayed and pined for her soldier husband. The Sunday after Christmas of 1861, Bettie Ann took up her pen to send him all the home news of churchgoing, hog raising, and Negro sales. The centerpiece of the letter was a sketch of their thirteen-month-old Joe, a whirlwind who was just then playing at her feet.

"Our little darling," she wrote, ". . . has improved a great deal in walking, and you would be pleased to see him running across the room which he does sometimes twenty times before he seems tired. He has a fashion of walking with his little hands laid upon his breast, which makes him totter a good deal. . . . [H]e eats as hearty as a little shoat."[2]

When the Civil War ended, the elder Dr. Kinyoun returned to practice medicine. His son would follow in his footsteps. Despite upheaval in family life—relocation to Centre View, Missouri, and the death of his mother when he was twelve—Joseph Kinyoun found his calling early as his father's apprentice. Following his training at St. Louis Medical College in Missouri, and then at Bellevue Hospital Medical College in New York, where he completed his M.D. in 1882, he returned to Missouri to join his father's medical practice.[3]

While at home in Centre View, he met a young Missourian named Susan Elizabeth Perry—Lizzie—and married her. They were both twenty-three. Within a year Lizzie bore a girl who died in childhood.[4]

While working with his father, Joseph Kinyoun started reading exciting reports about the French chemist Louis Pasteur, who was exploring the world of microbes. Through the lens of a microscope, Dr. Kinyoun immersed himself in the study of bacteria as agents of disease.

Kinyoun returned east with his bride to continue his study of bacteriology at Bellevue Hospital, and in 1886 he joined the U.S. Marine Hospital Service, the federal agency that inspected ships for disease, imposed maritime quarantines, and tended sick seamen. The service needed doctors like Kinyoun, with a passion for bacteriology, who could infuse service operations with the powerful new science. So the fledgling physician was asked to set up a bacteriology laboratory at the quarantine station in New York. It was in an unimposing one-room lab, up in the attic of the Marine Hospital on Staten Island, that he started to make his name.

A ship landed in New York Harbor with passengers racked by cramps and relentless diarrhea. Local clinicians feared the worst—cholera—but nobody knew for sure. The symptoms were variable and vague; they could mimic those of other diseases. It was Kinyoun's job to confirm it or rule it out. From the ailing passengers, he obtained samples and prepared slides. Squinting through the microscope lens, he saw a swarm of short, rod-shaped bacteria with hairy little fringes called flagellae, swimming around on the glass slide. It was *Vibrio cholerae,* the bacteria that causes cholera.

This was the first bacteriologic diagnosis of cholera in the United States, or anywhere in the western hemisphere.[5] At age twenty-seven, Joe Kinyoun was a force to reckon with.

In 1891, Kinyoun moved his one-room operation to Washington, D.C., to what came to be called the National Hygienic Laboratory, where he gained broad powers to pursue bacteriologic diagnoses of other epidemic diseases. Out of his slides and test tubes emerged the embryo of a vast biomedical research empire that decades later would become known as the National Institutes of Health.

But back in 1899, Kinyoun was simply helping America catch up with Europe, where the original microbe hunters, like Pasteur in France and Robert Koch in Germany, had begun the revolution in infectious disease study. Kinyoun now made a pilgrimage to the mecca of microbiology, studying at the Pasteur Institute in Paris and at Koch's laboratory in Berlin. From Koch he learned the classic protocol, essentially a recipe for how to prove a germ caused a disease: 1) isolate the germ from a patient; 2) grow the germ in pure culture; 3) inoculate the germ into a lab animal and reproduce the disease; and 4) isolate the identical germ from the test animal. A century later, this circle of proof would continue to govern the diagnosis of infectious diseases. He also learned how to make an antitoxin against diphtheria by harvesting disease-fighting antibodies from the blood of horses exposed to the germ.

When he returned to the National Hygienic Laboratory in the United States, Kinyoun brought with him the European techniques that helped to transform the practice of medical diagnosis, from the ancient bedside art of observing symptoms to a lab science using microscopes, cultures, stains, and slides. Symptoms like fever and pain could be vague and misleading. Bacteriology offered a way to test a diagnostic hypothesis. Its truths were verifiable; it had the beauty of certainty. Or so he thought.

Just after Kinyoun's National Hygienic Laboratory marked its first decade, his boss cut short his tenure and gave him a job far away. The supervising surgeon general of the Marine Hospital Service was Walter Wyman, a great gruff walrus of a man. A brusque bachelor, Wyman regarded the men of the corps as his family, and he was famed for abrupt transfers. He also regarded his primary mission as the imposition of the police powers of quarantine.[6] Now, quarantine duty was calling from the Pacific Coast, and he had Kinyoun in mind for the job.

With bubonic plague now ravaging China, Wyman rightly knew that the Pacific portal of the United States was vulnerable, so he enlisted Joseph Kinyoun to combat it. He told Kinyoun to pack up his family—which now included three children and a pregnant Lizzie—and go west.

Kinyoun was shocked by this abrupt transfer. After running the National Hygienic Laboratory, being sent back to police a port city against disease must have been a humiliating demotion. But Wyman had homed in on Kinyoun's replacement at the Hygienic Lab, so Kinyoun was California bound. Although Kinyoun was a brilliant bacteriologist, he was decidedly the wrong man for the job of quarantine officer on the Golden Gate. The port, a melting pot simmering with racial tensions, needed a doctor with a diplomat's touch. Instead, the city got an intellectually acute but autocratic scientist with a bruised ego who expected a level of deference the city wasn't prepared to give.

On the eve of Kinyoun's reluctant departure from Washington, D.C., his fellow physicians feted him with a farewell banquet at Rauscher's Restaurant. Their toasts were printed up in a cream-colored program bound with blue silk cord. Rumpled and stained from the night's festivities, a copy would rest with his papers until he died.

"Ah, happy, proud America! Thrice happy to possess men of Kinyoun's stamp, with all their faculties calmly and resolutely bent upon the fulfillment of a noble duty to mankind," intoned the toastmaster that night. "I wish you God-speed in your journey across the continent to the Golden Gate of the Pacific Ocean, where new fields of activity and new friends await you. . . ."[7]

After a week on the train with a pregnant wife and three small children, Kinyoun reached his foggy exile. Temporarily ensconced in the plush and gilt Palace Hotel, with its liveried doormen, he found rates that no health officer could afford. It was "the spider's trap for the eastern fly, and everyone pays tribute to these money sharks, on setting foot in San Francisco," he wrote to relatives and colleagues back East.[8]

He checked out. Kinyoun bundled his family into a carriage that clopped down Market Street to the Ferry Building, where they boarded the steamer *George Sternberg*. Five miles and forty minutes later, the boat swung into a sheltered inlet on the northern shore of Angel Island.

Facing north, away from San Francisco toward the tiny Marin County hamlet of Tiburon, his new headquarters was an eyesore in paradise. The biggest island in the bay, Angel Island was an ancient Miwok Indian camp, now occupied by U.S. quarantine and military officers. Its 740 acres were canopied with oak, madrone, bay laurel, and eucalyptus. Washed by the blue-green waters of Raccoon Strait, Hospital Cove might have made a beautiful spot for a resort hotel, Kinyoun mused. Then he beheld the primitive quarantine station and sparsely furnished cottage. His wife, Lizzie, was appalled. Kinyoun's heart sank.

The ramshackle wharf and quarantine station's dirt roads melted into mud rivulets in the rainy season. And if the quarantine officer's quarters were primitive, facilities for immigrants were even worse. There was no shed to shelter immigrants after their disinfecting bath. So the new arrivals had to stand, soaked and shivering, in the bay wind. It was a cold hygienic threshold to what would become in later years the Ellis Island of the Pacific Coast.

His new island home had few neighbors, no school, and little amusement for the children: Mary Alice, Conrad, Perry, and their new redheaded baby, John Nathan. There was a pier for fishing, but Kinyoun found Pacific fish to be insipid fare. Lizzie had a bad foot that kept her housebound. Too frail for more than one evening out in fourteen months, she was often in a raw temper.[9] They were isolated and made few friends. At night, it seemed that they were the ones in quarantine, bound by the sigh of the waves, the tolling of fog bells, and the pulse of the lighthouse.

The bright spot in their island exile was photography: Lizzie spent evenings in her darkroom, conjuring blurry portraits of her children out of the vinegary chemical bath. This hobby kept a kind of peace; Joseph had his lab, and Lizzie had hers.

Kinyoun chafed in the epaulets of his federal public health officer's uniform, which made him look ridiculous, he said, like a "major-domo" or a "government mule."[10] He'd been a young star in the Marine Hospital Service, nailing the cholera diagnosis while still in his twenties. Why had Dr. Wyman rewarded him with a transfer to this rude place, remote from the nerve center of public health? Kinyoun bitterly joked that Dr. Wyman had sent him out West to bury him. Writing to one of his mentors, Kinyoun swore that if that were the case, he would prove to be "a rather lively corpse."[11]

For certain, his scientific pedigree wasn't worth a wooden nickel in this rowdy town, where bankers, bosses, and broadsheets ruled. Kinyoun resented the grip of merchants on the life of the city and its public health. "You know," he wrote the folks back East, "San Francisco is frequently called 'Jew Town.' Well named."[12] He imagined that the city's Jewish businessmen were trying to get rid of him. About that, Kinyoun was wrong; *all* the city's businessmen wanted to get rid of him. His plague work was bad for business. The more the city reviled him, the more Kinyoun relished his image as the hero of a lonely public health crusade.

"I fortunately for one time in my life assumed the role of Dav[ey] Crockett . . . knowing that I was right," he confided to a friend.[13] Guarding the nation's health, he felt that he was under siege, much like his coonskin-capped hero in the Alamo.

One night, his wife, Lizzie, dreamed that the surgeon general came unannounced to Angel Island and requested a candle from her so he could inspect the quarantine station in the dark. Wait for my husband, she protested. What does it mean, Joe? she asked Kinyoun later. The surgeon general was in the dark, and he needed Kinyoun to light his way—it seemed clear enough. Kinyoun longed to be like his namesake, the biblical Joseph, honored by Pharaoh for his interpretation of the nightmare about to unfold on this alien coast.[14]

THE SPECTER OF PLAGUE had risen up before here. In June 1899, the Japanese steamship *Nippon Maru* had docked in San Francisco after two deaths at sea and two stowaways who jumped overboard with alleged plague ravaging their bodies. It had been impossible to prove the diagnosis. Indeed, Kinyoun's own lab analysis disputed it.

But now the memory of another ship haunted Kinyoun—the steamer *Australia,* which arrived from plague-stricken Honolulu in January 1900. It moored at the dock where the sewers from Chinatown emptied. The Chinese soon observed great numbers of rats dying on their roofs and in their courtyards. It seemed probable the rats had gained entrance to Chinese homes through the sewer pipes.[15]

Quarantine officers were always under pressure to grant ships a speedy permission to dock. Still, Kinyoun had always tried to be vigilant. In January 1900, he ordered ships coming from the infected zones of Hong Kong, Honolulu, Sydney, and Kobe to fly the yellow warning flag, the sign of a ship that has come from a plague port.

Kinyoun's letters to Dr. Wyman in Washington warning of the plague threat had grown increasingly shrill. He feared that inbound military ships from Manila might be capable of importing the plague into San Francisco. He thought the authorities overseas were concealing the risk.[16] Could he have missed something?

With Kellogg hovering at his side, Kinyoun peered through the microscope at the bacteria from Wong's tissues and blood. He felt a throb of recognition. Yes, this was it—the rose-tinted rods, dark at the ends. To be sure of his diagnosis, Kinyoun had to isolate it in pure culture and inoculate test animals to replicate the illness of Wong Chut King. After filling a syringe with bacteria from the dead man, he injected a rat, two guinea pigs, and a monkey. If the rod-shaped germs were plague bacteria, the animals would sicken. If they died with the same symptoms, he would biopsy their lymph nodes. If he found plague germs in their lymph fluid, he would have his proof. He placed the test animals back in their cages, and then inside large earthenware vessels for safety, and waited.

Kinyoun wired the first of a string of telegrams conveying the alarming news to Dr. Wyman in federal code, using strange phrases like "suspected bumpkin."[17]

Translated, the word *bumpkin* meant plague. Suspected plague in Chinatown. The encrypted messages eluded the Western Union operators and reporters hanging around the telegraph office. Singing over the wires, the messages traveled eastward over the cryptic signature of Kinyoun under his code name, "Abutment."

Downtown, the *San Francisco Chronicle* and other papers ridiculed the plague scare as a comic opera, a bubonic opera buffa. Political pundits believed the quarantine was a bit of jobbery staged to win funds and clout for the city's board of health. There were jokes about the "bubonic board of health." Kinyoun was branded a charlatan. The *San Francisco Bulletin* lampooned him in a rollicking rhyme:

> *Have you heard of the deadly bacillus,*
> *Scourge of a populous land,*
> *Bacillus that threatens to kill us,*
> *When found in a Chinaman's gland? . . .*

> *Well the monkey is living and thriving,*
> *The guinea pigs seem to be well,*
> *And the Health Board is vainly contriving*
> *Excuses for having raised . . .*[18]

Inside Chinatown, it *was* hell. Anxious, hungry, fearing for their lost wages and unattended jobs, the Chinese were sick with dread. Those who believed the disease was plague feared being trapped in the infected zone. Those who doubted that plague was real—by all accounts, the majority—feared that the quarantine was merely a pretext for more discrimination, a prelude to fire or demolition, imprisonment or detention. Discrimination was the bitter taste they swallowed with their daily rice, but who knew what new torments the whites might contrive? Outside the quarantine, whites chafed at the inconvenience of it all: Launderers, cooks, and laborers were absent from duty. Hostesses and hoteliers found meager pickings without their chefs and servants. Guests in downtown hostelries went hungry because kitchen staffs were trapped inside the barricades. Food, mail, and supplies were passed between the zones with difficulty or not at all.

After three days of quarantine, no new cases of the so-called plague had materialized. The test animals were still alive. Moreover, the Chinese were threatening to file a lawsuit protesting the blockade and asking for damages. The city health department now felt foolish and had no choice but to lift the quarantine.

Rumors of the blockade's end brought people pouring into the streets of Chinatown in anticipation of freedom. At four P.M. on March 10, the cordons came down and cheers went up. Thousands of Chinese flowed from the quarantined zone into greater San Francisco. Food deliveries recommenced. Men went back to work in hotels and kitchens all over town. Whites, too, cheered the end of their disrupted dinners. The *Examiner* published a celebratory verse.

THE RAISING OF THE QUARANTINE

Sweet Fong is at his post once more
And cooking reigns supreme;
Once more upon the kitchen range
A wealth of viands steam,
And joyful Plenty smiles again
Where Famine's hand was laid;
For, lo! The Board of Health has raised
The Chinatown blockade.[19]

But the poems and jokes, the cheers and celebration, were premature.

Two days later, on March 12, the scuffling and scrabbling animals inside the cages of the Angel Island lab went silent. When Kinyoun looked in, he found the rat and the guinea pigs lying cold in their cages. The monkey grew listless, hung his head, and died the next day.

The Boy from Catfish Creek

WHILE KINYOUN BROODED OVER his plague experiments on fog-bound Angel Island, another doctor kept watch over the sunstruck Mediterranean from his post in Genoa, Italy. If Kinyoun was a prodigy, thirty-two-year-old Rupert Lee Blue was a late bloomer just coming into flower. He too had recently been dispatched by the Marine Hospital Service to a remote lookout for epidemics. On June 27, 1900, Blue picked up a local newspaper and read a report that made his pulse quicken: A dozen people had fallen sick and three were dead of bubonic plague in Greece and Turkey. He dashed off a dispatch to Washington.

"The bubonic pest is slowly marching Northward along the Levantine shore and invading Europe from the East," he wrote to the surgeon general.[1] His prediction of an epidemic storming the gates of Europe was grippingly phrased to catch the eye of his boss, Walter Wyman, but it turned out to be a false alarm. A dozen cases on the Aegean coast didn't herald the return of the Black Death to Europe.

Still, Blue was right to be on the alert. Since biblical times, plague had sown death around the world in sweeping pandemics—super-epidemics—three times over two millennia. As a Sunday schooler, Blue had no doubt read the Book of Samuel's passage about a plague among the Philistines, who suffered "emerods in their secret parts," a poetic description of the signature symptom—buboes, or swollen glands, in the hollows of the groin and armpits that give the disease its name. In the sixth century, Justinian's Plague took nearly one hundred million lives in Asia, Africa, and Europe. In the fourteenth century, the plague pandemic known as the Black Death killed fifty million victims, including a quarter of Europe's population. Aftershocks were felt for centuries, in outbreaks like the great plague of London in 1665.

Now, the third plague pandemic, centered in Hong Kong in 1894, was spreading along the trade routes. While plague once traveled on the wind that drove sailing ships, it now migrated at twentieth-century speed aboard new coal-fired steamships.[2]

Its symptoms were violent: Rampant fever, crushing headache, overwhelming nausea, and profound weakness swept over a person who had been strong only hours before. Inflamed lymph glands struggled to contain the invading bacteria. Wherever they swelled, a painful red bubo erupted. Inky hemorrhages burst from small vessels, staining the skin with blue-black tattoos—the fearful "tokens" of Black Death. The pulse galloped at first, then later dwindled to a thread dancing beneath the doctor's finger. Delirium and pain unhinged the mind and stirred the limbs in an agitated dance of death. Victims in their final agony plucked at the bedclothes, unable to bear the slightest touch on their swellings.

Plague's only mercy was its speedy end. When buboes were the main symptom, plague killed in five days. If a victim was spitting blood, a symptom of plague in the lungs, death came in two or three days. So-called pneumonic plague was the rarest and deadliest form of the disease. It was also the only form now known to be contagious, spread from person to person by saliva as the coughing victims helplessly infected caretakers and family. Bubonic or pneumonic, it all started from the same germ, the bacteria known, variously, as *Bacillus pestis* and *Yersinia pestis*.

More terrible than the scourge itself was the effect it had on the psyche: It turned humans into beasts. Giovanni Boccaccio gives an eyewitness account of plague-stricken Florence in his preface to *The Decameron,* describing how the sick were abandoned in agony, corpses layered in mass graves, and princely palaces left empty:

> . . . [T]hings had reached the point where the dying received
> no more consideration than the odd goat would today. . . . As

there was not sufficient consecrated ground in which to bury the vast number of corpses that arrived at every church day after day and practically hour by hour . . . enormous pits were dug in graveyards, once saturation point had been reached, and the new arrivals were dropped into these by the hundred; here they were packed in layers, the way goods are stowed in a ship's hold, and each layer would get a thin layer of earth until the pit was filled up.[3]

Daniel Defoe, writing of seventeenth-century London in his 1722 work, *A Journal of the Plague Year,* said that the terror of the epidemic prompted "knavery and collusion" in infected towns where officials falsified burial records and fearful people hid the sick and the dead.

. . . [A]ll that could conceal their distempers did it, to prevent their neighbors shunning and refusing to converse with them, and also to prevent authority shutting up their houses; which, though it was not yet practised, yet was threatened, and people were extremely terrified at the thoughts of it.[4]

Doctors were powerless to halt the Black Death, but that didn't inhibit their invention of strange nostrums. To ward off infected vapors, they prescribed smelling apples, molded from sandalwood, pepper, camphor, and rose. People drank infusions of treacle, wine, and minced snake, while the rich took costlier compounds of crushed pearls and molten gold. One Italian apothecary named Gentile da Foligno crafted fanciful remedies from gemstones—including amethyst amulets and potions of powdered emerald. The latter remedy was said to be "so potent that, if a toad looked at it, its eyes would crack."[5] Unfortunately for the desperate rich, ingesting gems and gold didn't cure plague and may even have hastened their death.

From fourteenth-century Italy, too, came ancient protocols for plague control: lazarettos, or isolation hospitals named after Lazarus, the leprous beggar in the biblical parable; and *la quarantina,* the quarantine of ships, originally set at forty days to commemorate Christ's sojourn in the wilderness.[6]

Given the dearth of scientific knowledge, people wrapped plague in religious mystery and interpreted its hideous effects as God's punishment. To explain its occurrence, some people wove myths about plague showering down from comets, spread house to house by she-demons or flowing from wells poisoned by Jews. The scapegoats were bricked up in their homes and burned alive by suspicious and vengeful villagers. Such myths made plague a metaphor for medical catastrophe, while the reality of its transmission—from the bite of a lowly rat flea—remained veiled in mystery.

By the late nineteenth century, those remedies were consigned to history. But the Victorian Age introduced some harrowing remedies of its own. British colonial physicians in India prescribed that plague patients drink diluted carbolic acid, or cool their fevers by taking a refreshing ice-water enema.[7]

Despite Blue's premonition of doom in Genoa, the Black Death didn't renew a major assault on Europe in June 1900. But the suspected Mediterranean cases kept him on alert for new waves of the third plague pandemic, then migrating from China across the sea to other ports around the world. Plague had inflicted violent mortality in Hong Kong, and Washington was monitoring reports by the British colonial authorities. From that day in Italy onward, plague would be a leitmotif in Blue's career. Within the year, he would be ordered to return from Italy to the United States and assigned to San Francisco, where the infection was just beginning to insinuate itself into the city.

Like his predecessor Joseph Kinyoun, Rupert Blue was a son of the South. Born in Richmond County, North Carolina, he moved at the age of three to his mother's hometown of Marion, South Carolina. His father, like Kinyoun's, had served in the Civil War. Unlike Kinyoun, who entered public health work as a pioneer bacteriologist and founder of a prestigious national laboratory, Blue started as a simple foot soldier in the war on disease. He was a soldier's son, drawn to a life in uniform, but when he enlisted in the U.S. Marine Hospital Service, it was not as a warrior, but as a healer.

Descended from a line of Carolina Scotsmen who stood over six feet tall, Blue had blue eyes, jet hair, and a barrel-chested Victorian frame well upholstered by a robust appetite and a love of boxing. He styled his hair with a center part and grew a curved handlebar mustache that he twirled when amused or twisted when preoccupied. He was the sixth of eight children—three boys and five girls—born to Colonel John Gilchrist Blue and his wife, Annie Maria Evans. His grandparents owned spacious Carolina plantations with many slaves.[8] However, Rupert Blue, born on May 30, 1868, was a child of the Reconstruction and lived amid freed servants and field hands. Within their conservative southern milieu, the Blues were more progressive than many of their contemporaries. Mrs. Blue had been one of the few girls in the antebellum South to go to college. Colonel Blue, for his part, practiced law and served in the South Carolina State Legislature, where he championed the cause of women's education. His lonely campaign drew jibes that he sought to see women admitted to South Carolina's famous military academy, the Citadel.[9] His bill failed, but a century later, the joke it inspired would come true.

The Blue boys and girls—Sallie, Effie, Ida, William, Victor, Rupert, Kate Lilly, and Henriette—toiled in Marion's public and private schools, studying history and Latin. Of the younger Blues, Victor and Kate were extroverts who sparkled in company, while Rupert and Henriette (called Henriet or Hettie for short) were both shy, indwelling souls whom folks found it easy to underestimate. Rupert read avidly about classical Rome, studied the Bible, and devoured accounts of Napoleon.

The Blue children were baptized and confirmed in the white-pillared Presbyterian church on Main Street. They straddled logs on the reed-choked banks of Catfish Creek, less than a mile from their back door, to angle for pikes, jacks, and catfish. There were quail and partridge for the hunting. The boys' menagerie included blooded calves and purebred dogs, Angora goats and merino sheep, while the girls kept pedigreed cats and prize poultry.

In spring, they held contests to identify the first notes of birdsong from the chuck-will's-widows in the Carolina pines. The most succulent treat of a summer morning was savored in stealth. Creeping into the melon patch at dawn, with the dew still on the vines, the Blue children would "bust melons" open with their fists, devouring the ruby centers without ceremony or silverware.[10]

The family's plantation, Bluefields, was a stout, unpretentious family farmhouse with a broad-railed porch and heart-of-pine floors that rang with the steps of the parents and their eight growing offspring. On three hundred acres around their plantation, the family raised tobacco and cotton, corn and lumber.

Marion County, South Carolina, is shaped like a pork chop, stuck in the fork of the Big and Little Pee Dee Rivers. In summer, it is steamed languidly by a swamp that local Indians called Withlacoochee, but which the children knew simply as Catfish Creek. The town of Marion is anchored by stately Greek revival mansions, fringed with purple wisteria and the fuchsia blooms of crape myrtle. Any passing Yankees who dared steal its gray-green swags of Spanish moss as souvenirs would be bitten by red bugs, a source of local mirth to this day.

Marion was named for Francis Marion, the "Swamp Fox" of the Revolutionary War, who eluded the British and survived on roots and water. A century later, the boy who staged naval battles in Catfish Creek identified as much with the heroes of the Revolutionary War as with those of the War Between the States. As the Civil War waned, Marion escaped Sherman's torch by an accident of the weather: A rainstorm flooded the Pee Dee River, and its rising waters deflected the Union general's attack. Thankful Marionites dubbed the river "Sherman's freshet."[11] Rupert Blue was born a son of the Confederacy, but he aspired to be in the Sons of the Revolution.

It's often said the hero displayed gifts of brilliance and leadership in childhood. But, plainly, Rupert Blue didn't start out as Marion's most illustrious son. That honor belonged to his brother Victor, two years older, who emulated his father's military service by entering the Naval Academy at Annapolis. After graduation, Victor served with distinction in the Spanish-American War, where he performed dangerous surveillance, gathering intelligence on enemy ships in the port of Santiago, Cuba. For this, he was feted as a naval hero. Chiseled, gallant, graceful in society, Victor cast a long shadow over his little brother. Round, shy, halting in public, the younger brother nicknamed "Pert" got lost in the glare of Victor's glamour.[12]

Victor was "the family paragon, and entirely worthy of the great love his parents, brothers and sisters bore him," his sister Kate Lilly rhapsodized. About her other brother, she measured her words.[13]

"There was the greatest difference between Victor and Rupert," Kate said. When Victor returned home a war hero, he "hob-nobed with everybody he had ever known," she said. The younger boy was neither war hero nor socialite. "Rupert is very different," Kate said. "He just cannot stand on the street corner and give the glad hand to to somebody he might have gone to school with. . . ."[14]

After school days were over, Rupert got his first taste of medicine in 1888, when he spent a precollege year studying practical pharmacy in Latta, South Carolina, a tiny hamlet eleven miles north of his home. He lived in a boardinghouse and was desperately homesick for the plantation but put on a brave face. "Thanks to a nature that is cosmopolitan," he wrote gamely, "I am content to live anywhere."[15] Truth was, he so craved contact that he sent stamps home to coax the family to write him letters.

Blue's boyhood ended abruptly one winter night. Although he stood a robust six feet two, Rupert's father wasn't as strong as he looked. During the Civil War, while leading a regiment called the Scotch boys, he managed to dodge lead balls and cannonfire, only to carry home scars in his heart, possibly from rheumatic fever. Although he was a noted temperance leader who abstained from alcohol, he indulged freely in tobacco, which further strained his heart. Even getting about the farm became difficult, and his sons implored him to rest. That winter, his vigor failed utterly. He left the clinging damp of Marion for the brisk air of his old home in Richmond County, North Carolina. Victor, then on naval exercises in Europe, and Rupert, at his pharmacy in Latta, wrote anxious letters home, begging for news of "Pa's" recovery. When Mrs. Blue and the girls opened Colonel Blue's letters home, they saw a frail and spidery hand that crawled across the page, belying his words of stout cheer and sure recovery.[16]

On Christmas Day 1888, Colonel Blue suffered a heart attack. He lingered through the New Year. As his family gathered around his bed late on Sunday night, January 6, 1889, he died. They buried him in North Carolina.[17]

His widow was left to manage on her own with two teenage girls at home—Kate and Hettie. Her eldest son, Bill, would manage the farm. Her middle son would continue his naval career. Her youngest boy, a twenty-year-old pharmacy apprentice, had no degree and meager prospects. That would change fast.

Galvanized by his family's loss, Rupert now entered the University of Virginia at Charlottesville—"Mr. Jefferson's University." He wanted to reassure the family that, despite the enticements of college life, his soul wasn't in jeopardy.

"You must not fear for my morals because I can not be persuaded to do a thing, when that thing is distasteful to me. I will not assimilate the vices of others," he wrote to Kate. "[I]f I am spared to good health I can accomplish something, for I have the will & ambition."[18]

After two years of study in the serpentine-walled campus at Charlottesville, Rupert entered medical school at the University of Maryland, Baltimore. There, he wasn't the most brilliant student, but rather an earnest toiler with a sharp new sense of duty.

"I am working like a Trojan," he wrote to Kate, "and I trust that my labors will be rewarded." Money was tight since his father's death, and he had to choose between tuition and travel. "I may come home in the spring," he wrote, but he added, "It depends entirely on the state of my exchequer. I want enough to take a short course in hospital diagnosis." In his command of medicine, he feared he was falling behind another Virginia school chap and friendly rival, Joe Guthrie, who surpassed him by taking a hospital course in New York. "There is," he despaired, "so much to learn. . . ."[19]

There were distractions. While he toiled, "matrimonial fever" swept the country cotillions of Marion. Rupert had been courting a local belle named Miss Emily, but he was a diffident suitor and wrote of love as a recurrent affliction from which "I hope I will be cured. . . ."[20]

Finally, Blue's medical school travails paid off. He won a rank of second place in anatomy class, with an average of 90 percent in other subjects.

On April 15, 1892, Blue graduated from medical school. None of his family attended his graduation, so he wrote a letter sketching the pageantry for his absent kin.

"Our commencement exercises yesterday were pompous and ceremonious to an extreme," he wrote.

"I begin my professional career today with perfect cognizance of the many responsibilities which rest upon my shoulders," he said. "When I listened to the valedictory address, I mentally determined that I should ever be found on the side of right—let the consequences be as they may. That temptation no matter how alluring should not deter me from the path of rectitude," he went on. But anticipating that Kate would mock his solemnity, he rushed to add, "This confession may seem strange to you, knowing my early training and fixed attributes of character; but I will reply by saying that a physician's life is one beset with peculiar environments and open to many possible indictments."

Then, trying out his new title, he signed the letter with a professional flourish:

"Love to all. Yours, R. L. Blue, M.D."[21]

After an internship in Baltimore, where he treated sick oystermen, R. L. Blue, M.D., applied to join the U.S. Marine Hospital Service, the guardian of ports and quarantines that during his tenure would grow into the U.S. Public Health Service. Admission to the service was granted by a competitive exam covering medical and general academic knowledge. Blue was nervous. Kate, now an aspiring librarian, sent a shipment of great books so he could stuff his head with learned allusions. They came too late. But Rupert made a good show, reading Latin fluently. Still, entrance into the Marine Hospital Service commissioned corps required a presidential appointment and confirmation by the Senate. There were twenty-five applicants and only four vacancies.

As he waited for word, he gnawed away his anxiety by indulging in his father's vice—tobacco—and wrote letters to his family.

"This branch of the service has many advantages over the Navy or Army. . . . I am in exactly the same straits that Victor was in that summer he was home from the 2 years' cruise, [i.e.] in awaiting orders," he wrote Kate. "I do not know yet where I will be permanently located. It can be anywhere from Maine to California or from the Lakes to the Gulf. There is some excitement in this condition and I am making tobacco fly. . . .

"Our uniforms are the same as the Naval. The rank of assistant surgeon in the [Marine Hospital Service] is that of a lieutenant, the pay is from 16 to 17 to 18 hundred per year. You see the pay is better than that of an Ensign or [Lieutenant] on shore duty. But of course there are some disadvantages, viz. being ordered to a yellow fever quarantine station at Key West, Fla., or the Dry Tortugas. Tell Ma and Sallie not to fret. . . ."[22]

Joking years later about his choice of public health over private practice, he told his mother that private physicians were too dependent upon the money and the gratitude of rich patients. And gratitude, he said, is part of the disease: Once the patient's cured, it goes away. But the truth was, he didn't aspire to just cure disease. He wanted to *prevent* it entirely.[23]

To Blue's relief, his appointment to the U.S. Marine Hospital Service was promptly confirmed. One of his first assignments sent him south to the humid seaport of Galveston, Texas. There, in the Gulf town, he gave his mother a new cause to fret—not yellow fever, but a fever common to young men. Across the footlights of a Galveston theater, he saw a vivacious young actress and was smitten. Her name was Juliette Downs, and she was the daughter of a southern railroad man. Her choice of a stage career would have upset many a good Victorian matriarch, especially one born of genteel southern stock like Annie Maria Blue. One might court an actress, even sow a few wild oats. But marriage? An actress was certainly a questionable candidate for daughter-in-law.

Victor, on the other hand, displayed the same impeccable taste in a mate as he had in a career. Eleanor Foote Stuart, called "Nellie," was a cameo blond beauty with a halo of curls and the daughter of a military family of means. Victor and Nellie produced two handsome sons, traveled the world, and returned home often to bask in the adoration of Marion society. Today, no one in the town of Marion—where everyone knew the Blues—even recalls hearing of a visit by Rupert's love, Juliette.

Bucking convention, Rupert and Juliette were wed in 1895 and, after a stop in New York, soon headed for his assignments on the West Coast. The newly wed assistant surgeon in the Marine Hospital Service was stationed at the Angel Island quarantine station in San Francisco Bay, boarding ships, peering into dark and pungent cargo holds, and checking passengers from stateroom to steerage. In his performance reviews, Blue's supervising officers rated him highly for his "diligence, discretion, and tact" and for solid professionalism, but they also noted that he liked an occasional drink and was "somewhat disposed to be hurried."[24]

At twenty-seven, with his country boyhood behind him, Blue had to think about supporting a stylish wife with a taste for the finer things. In the rainy season, Angel Island turned into a mudslide, so the Blues moved into a hotel in the city. But the lifestyle there proved to be expensive. Rupert still sent home a portion of his paycheck as a monthly allowance for his widowed mother and his two unmarried sisters, Kate and Henriet. It was difficult to manage on $1,800 a year.

When the hospital service posted him to Italy in 1900, Rupert and Juliette reveled in an Easter holiday in Rome—accompanied by

Juliette's mother, Mrs. Downs. Juliette and her mother explored modern Rome, where Giacomo Puccini was following up his opera *La Bohème* with a new work called *Tosca*. On his own, Rupert explored *la città eterna*, wandering wide-eyed through the Forum, studying the classical antiquities he knew from school and the early Christian relics he recalled from his Bible lessons. He wrote to his mother and Kate to implore them to make a return pilgrimage with him. Juliette's father, who had once done a favor for a touring Italian cleric, arranged a papal audience. The aging Pope Leo XIII clasped the young couple in benediction. As a lifelong Presbyterian, Blue was skeptical, but something happened when the pontiff took his face in his hands and, speaking in French, blessed Blue's mother in her faraway farmhouse. "I like this grand old prelate," Blue admitted, completely won over.[25]

After Italy, the return to domestic assignments would seem dull to any couple in their twenties: Portland had no Puccini, and Milwaukee had no Michelangelo. Money was tight, and Rupert continued to send a portion of every paycheck home—which meant less for ball gowns, carriages, dining, and nights out. The life of a circuit-riding doctor strained the best of marriages. The romance kindled in the heat of Galveston and stoked by the *dolce vita* of Italy would be tested by the deep freeze of Milwaukee winters and the dreary rains of Portland.

Rupert lacked Victor's knack for military honors, social graces, and making an advantageous marriage. All too aware of his deficiency, he would season his brotherly love for Victor with rivalry all his life. Years later, when applying for membership in the Sons of the Revolution, he explained to Kate, "Victor has so many medals I wish to own a few badges myself in order to make a fair showing in uniform beside him."[26] Although Rupert Blue was no soldier, he had subtler strengths that lay quiescent, waiting to be tested in a time of epidemic.

In his earliest surviving portrait as a working physician, Rupert appears every inch a warrior. He is dressed in the rich regalia of the Marine Hospital Service's dress uniform. His double-breasted frock coat of midnight blue was lined with eighteen gilt buttons and topped by gold-braided shoulder boards. His belt was vellum, shot with gold wire and striped with navy and gold silk. From it hung a thirty-inch ceremonial sword, with a white sharkskin grip wrapped in gilt wire and adorned with a heavy golden tassel. The service supplied a twenty-five-page pamphlet to outline all of its magnificent tailoring details, down to every last anchor and eagle ornament.[27]

In his dress uniform, Rupert Blue looked almost as much a military man as his brother Victor. Only the gilded clasp on his belt buckle hinted at a different mission. Engraved on its face was the anchor of the Marine Hospital Service, signifying the seamen who were his first patients. It also bears a caduceus, a winged wand with twin serpents interlaced. The caduceus was a symbol of both maritime commerce and the art of medicine. The caduceus also resembles the staff of Aesculapius, the progenitor of public health guardians. In ancient mythology, Aesculapius was a physician who outraged the gods by daring to bring the dead back to life. For his presumption, the god Zeus struck him down with a lightning bolt. Blue would later learn that a doctor could rattle politicians almost as much as Aesculapius had riled the gods.[28]

Nearly every day for the next two decades, Blue would live in the plain khaki fatigues of the hospital service's working uniform. But it was in full ceremonial regalia that he posed that day. Turning right in a heroic three-quarter profile, chin up and arms akimbo, he gazed with a look both dreamy and defiant toward a future he could not imagine.[29]

Hiding the Dead

JOSEPH KINYOUN GRASPED his proof defiantly. With stains and slides, with microscopes and the mute testimony of dead lab animals, he had identified the germ that killed Wong Chut King.

The killer, he now knew, was the same bacteria that had ravaged Asia and Europe since biblical times. Was this the beginning of an epidemic like the one described in *The Decameron,* one that would send rich and poor to common graves and leave Nob Hill mansions as vacant as Florentine palaces?

Although plague had ravaged Europe for thousands of years, its true nature and cause weren't discovered until 1894, after a feverish scientific race. Even after the bacterium was identified, how it entered the human body remained a mystery.

In 1894, as bubonic plague inflicted suffering and death on China, two rival scientists, Alexandre Yersin of Paris and Shibasaburo Kitasato of Tokyo, went to Hong Kong to identify the cause of plague. Both were eminent scientists, disciples of the pioneering microbe hunters Robert Koch, who identified the tuberculosis bacterium, and Louis Pasteur, who created the rabies vaccine. Yersin and Kitasato both used a basic technique in their work called Gram's stain.

The brainchild of a Danish scientist, Hans Christian Joachim Gram, the test cleverly exploits the tendency of different bugs to either soak up or shed certain colored dyes. Whereas growing colonies of bacteria in culture takes days to complete, testing the Gram's stain takes just minutes and requires only a few vials of blue or pink dye. A scientist drenches a sample of bacteria with blue dye, then rinses it. If the blue dye sticks, the germs are classified as "Gram positive." If the blue dye washes off and the germs instead absorb a second, pink-tinted dye, they are considered "Gram negative." Some well-known bacteria, such as staphylococcus and streptococcus, turn blue—Gram positive. But plague bacteria shed the blue dye and stain vivid pink—Gram negative. The staining pattern also highlights the distinctive features and shape of a bacterium: The rod-shaped plague bacteria turn deep rose at the rounded tips, so that they resemble closed safety pins.

In their haste to discover plague, however, the rival scientists Kitasato and Yersin announced different results of the Gram's stain. Kitasato was first to declare his results and rushed to tell the world that the plague bacteria stained blue—Gram positive. Later he vacillated, saying he didn't know.

Yersin arrived in Hong Kong four days after his rival. Lacking the authority to perform autopsies in the major hospital, he had to improvise. Working in a tent behind his straw hut, he paid British soldiers doing undertaker duty for access to bodies awaiting burial. After opening their coffins and dusting the lime off their bodies, Yersin biopsied their glands and found "a veritable puree of microbes."[1] Once purified and tested with the Gram's stain, the plague bacteria turned pink—Gram negative. Yersin had found the right answer.

To this day, Kitasato's blunder is baffling. Some historians speculate that he used a biopsy sample that was accidentally contaminated with staph or strep germs, which stained blue.

Though Kitasato and Yersin are usually credited as codiscoverers of the plague bacterium, it was Yersin's discovery that prevailed and prompted a name change from *Bacillus pestis* to *Yersinia pestis*. The landmark discovery gave scientists all over the world a way to identify the deadly germ.[2]

Just a baby germ in evolutionary terms, *Yersinia pestis* is now thought to be anywhere from 1,500 to 20,000 years old. It evolved from an ancient bacterium known as *Yersinia pseudotuberculosis*, a bug between 400,000 and 1.9 million years old that causes intestinal distress. From this benign parent, a germ of staggering virulence was born, one that when left untreated remains the most lethal bacterium known to humankind. Even today, when doctors have the curative antibiotic drugs that were undiscovered in 1900, bubonic plague is still evolving and springing surprises on the unsuspecting physician. In 1995, a drug-resistant strain of bubonic plague sickened a patient in Madagascar. Fortunately, alert scientists and doctors saved this patient with a sulfa drug combination to which the bug ultimately succumbed. But to shaken scientists, the message was clear: Plague is still active worldwide, one of many contenders in the global contest for microbial supremacy.[3]

Yersin's discovery gave Joseph Kinyoun's culprit a face and a fast tool with which to identify it. There were other tests, too: On culture plates, colonies of plague look like ground glass. And he applied Koch's postulates to prove that the plague germ had in fact killed Wong Chut King. First he isolated the bacteria. Then he grew them in pure culture. He injected the germs into lab animals. When the animals died of the same disease, he isolated the germ again, and voilà, he had apprehended the killer—bubonic plague.

But to the San Francisco citizen of 1900—even to most practicing physicians—the new bacteriology was still a form of black magic: mysterious, dimly understood, untrustworthy, and inferior to the laying on of hands and the observation of symptoms at the bedside. Fevers and swollen glands could signify anything from strep to syphilis, they said. Many practicing physicians in town dismissed the bacteriologist Kinyoun, and most folks trusted their family doctors.[4]

Newspapers lampooned the plague cleanup. Cartoonists sketched doctors plucking germs off Chinese scrolls. The bacteria were depicted as grinning, gargoyle-faced tadpoles. Caricatures of pigtailed immigrants were shown fleeing town. And on March 14, the *San Francisco Call* newspaper published a mock obituary, reporting the death of "A. Monk—At the Angel Island bubonic germ stock farm."

No one was more skeptical than Ng Poon Chew, the Presbyterian minister who founded and edited Chinatown's leading newspaper, the *Chung Sai Yat Po,* or *East-West Daily.* In his story announcing the results of the plague test, he spoke for an entire community that feared not so much that they would die from plague, but that they would be ruined by it:

THE MONKEY IS DEAD

. . . Alas, why should Chinatown's good name depend on the life and death of a monkey? If this monkey lived, then Chinatown would be exempt from fear and the Chinese would rejoice at the news. We don't know the implications of the English-language press commentary, and whether they are rooting for Chinatown or the monkey. We don't know whether luck will favor the physician or Chinatown. But this morning, the monkey was reported to be dead. In the view of this newspaper, the monkey's death was not caused by plague. Alas, the monkey's death was due to starvation—a result of its unlucky encounter with this physician.[5]

Rumors multiplied like bacteria. It was said the quarantine officer had poisoned the test animals to justify his diagnosis. Besides, everyone from Chinatown to Nob Hill believed that injecting fluid from the glands of a corpse—any corpse—could kill you. It was the liquid of putrefaction, not the germs of plague, that was causing death. All agreed that bacteriology was a ghoulish practice.

Daily headlines declared it a fraud. THE PLAGUE A PHANTOM: MORE BOUFFE BUSINESS BY THE HEALTH BOARD, the *Chronicle* railed on March 13. The next day, the paper proclaimed: NO PLAGUE IS FOUND. By St. Patrick's Day, with the town in a holiday mood, the paper concluded: BUBONIC SCARE HAS COLLAPSED.

In a counterpoint to the drumbeat of denial, a careful listener could hear the hammers in the coffin shops of Chinatown. On March 15, just one week after the death of Wong Chut King, a twenty-two-year-old laborer died on Sacramento Street. The next victim was a thirty-five-year-old cook, who died on March 17 on Dupont Street. The day after that, a middle-aged workingman collapsed and died on the tiny crooked alley called Oneida Place. All three had the plague stigmata on them.[6]

The politicians, the merchants, and the Chinese all had good reason for denying the diagnosis. No one wanted to see the yellow flag of pestilence flying over the portal to the Golden State. It would tarnish tourism and trade. It would turn Chinatown into a quarantine zone and subject the Chinese to the interventions of white doctors with their dissection tools, chemicals, and fire. To the Chinese, who were not unacquainted with epidemics, the cure must have seemed far worse than the disease.

But down at City Hall, San Francisco's mayor indulged the health board. James Duval Phelan was a Democratic reformer sandwiched between corrupt and boss-ridden mayors, but he was also an arch-enemy of Chinese immigration. And as the Chinese Exclusion Act of 1882 was coming up for renewal, the plague scare gave him another reason to sound off on the yellow peril posed by "coolies." Chinese labor had been sweet enough to railroad tycoons during the building of the transcontinental railroad, but with the dawn of the new century, a labor surplus frayed California's welcome mat. Phelan viewed Asian workers as a threat to the sons of the Golden State, even though many were native-born San Franciscans. Phelan would later run for the U.S. Senate under the slogan "Keep California White."[7]

So when Chinese consul Ho Yow threatened to sue the city for $500,000 to recover Chinatown's damages from the quarantine, Phelan's true feelings erupted:

"As to objections and suits by the Chinese, I desire to say that they are fortunate, with the unclean habits of their coolies and their filthy hovels, to be permitted to remain within the corporate limits of any American city," the mayor exploded. "In an economic sense, their presence has been, and is, a great injury to the working classes, and in a sanitary sense, they are a constant menace to the public health."[8]

Meanwhile, Consul Ho struggled to improve the quality of life for his people. He joined with the Chinese Six Companies in founding the new Oriental Dispensary at 828 Sacramento Street. An emergency hospital staffed with a mix of Western physicians and traditional Chinese herbalists, it was equipped with $1,500 in supplies bought with donations. The dispensary aimed to replace an old institution, the so-called halls of tranquillity, where destitute Chinese went to die.

In Washington, D.C., Surgeon General Walter Wyman prescribed a mass vaccination of all the Chinese in Chinatown. The product was a broth of heat-killed bacteria, called the Haffkine vaccine after its creator, Waldemar Haffkine, a Russian scientist who fled his homeland for a post at the Pasteur Institute in Paris. Haffkine's vaccine used the traditional technique of sparking protection by using a small amount of bacteria to arouse an immune reaction. The trouble was, it also provoked severe side effects, ranging from pain and swelling to fever and malaise and, occasionally, death. When it worked, its protection was short-lived. In people already exposed to the plague, the vaccine was extremely dangerous because it accelerated the germ's lethal attack. With such risks widely known, the vaccine was violently unpopular in Chinatown. Still, Wyman shipped almost two thousand doses of vaccine west the day after Wong Chut King died. He promised to send thirteen thousand more within two days and, after that, a stream of ten thousand doses a week.[9]

Wyman also sent three hundred bottles of Yersin's plague antiserum, a completely different product. The antiserum was a solution of antibodies, drawn from the blood of horses that had been exposed to plague. The antiserum could serve as a ready-made immune defense against infection, and it was safer than the vaccine for people already exposed to the plague. However, the antiserum was scarce and costly. Because its manufacture required horses, it was much more difficult and expensive to produce than a colony of bacteria that could simply be grown in a test tube. So the antiserum was used sparingly, and much of it was reserved for the doctors working in the midst of an outbreak.

While urging the mass vaccination—"Haffkinization"—of Chinatown, the surgeon general downplayed the dangers of the situation. He portrayed the measures as necessary simply to keep plague from establishing a base in the city and causing repeated outbreaks throughout the year.[10]

The *Examiner,* the newspaper owned by William Randolph Hearst, broke ranks with the other San Francisco papers, which ridiculed or denied plague outright. The *Examiner* saw the plague as a news opportunity. Enterprising reporter J. A. Boyle rolled up his sleeves and filed a first-person account of what it felt like to be injected with the Haffkine vaccination.

"The inoculation itself is entirely painless. . . . Within two hours, however, the serum had spread through my system and its effects began to be felt," wrote the journalistic guinea pig. "Shooting pains, slight at first, began near the point of injection and extended across the chest, down the arm and even up into my neck and head. My left arm felt numb and I moved it with difficulty. The muscles covering my shoulder blade felt as if they were being drawn together as by a rubber band," he added. "I was slightly dizzy, there was a ringing in my ears and I felt I was drifting into a stupor from which I did not particularly care to rouse myself. All this time, the pain in my shoulder, chest, neck and arm had been increasing until it was quite severe. I was unable to concentrate my mind and felt flushed and feverish."[11] Eight hours later, Boyle's pain eased, his head cleared, and his fever dropped. His ordeal was over, his story a success. But the stunt did nothing to convince those in Chinatown to roll up their sleeves.

By now, the mere sight of white health officers with their needles was enough to prompt a panic. Some whites who worked in Chinatown, like Donaldina Cameron, director of the Presbyterian Mission Home in Chinatown, attributed fear of the plague vaccine to superstition. She tried to encourage immunization, but the Chinese knew the Haffkine vaccine could sicken or even kill. A few mission girls lined up. One girl broke from the line, dashed to a second-story window, and jumped. Onlookers saw a flash of jacket and a wisp of black hair, and she disappeared. A thud sounded from below, where the girl was alive but in agony, crumpled on the sidewalk with smashed ankle-bones.[12]

A Presbyterian missionary of Scottish descent, Miss Cameron had one passionate calling: to rescue slave girls and prostitutes from servitude in Chinatown and convert them to Christianity. Sallying forth in her shirtwaists with leg-of-mutton sleeves, her auburn pompadour anchored by prim veiled hats, she raided vice cribs like Carry Nation with a Scots burr. The Chinese, skeptical of her meddling, called her *Fan Quai*, "White Devil." To her wards she was *Lo Mo*, or "Old Mother."[13]

One day while the quarantine was in effect, a nine-year-old girl named Ah Ching had come seeking help at the mission for her sister, who was dying of plague. Cameron shed her Victorian gown for Chinese pants, hid her russet head under an umbrella, and slipped past the quarantine lines.

After ascending through a skylight, she hopped roof to roof and found Ah Ching's boardinghouse. The girl was abandoned and slumped on a wooden chair out on the sidewalk. Miss Cameron carried her to the mission and summoned a doctor. In a surprising turn of events, the physician diagnosed not plague, but appendicitis. She died three hours later, victim of a burst appendix and of neglect spawned by plague phobia.[14]

Over Chinatown, columns of smoke rose from the bonfires of refuse that burned on Pacific Street. Plumbing was flushed with chemicals, masking the scent of cookery and crowded humanity with stinging clouds of disinfectant vapors. Mounds of white lime powder were scattered in chalky drifts against the balconied apartments, storefronts, and courtyards, so that the district looked like a Sierra village after a snowstorm. An oppressive stench hung over the district.

Downtown, the board of health met with the Chinese consul and the Chinese Six Companies, wrangling over details of the Chinatown cleanup of plague. All they could agree on was the need to clear out basements and dispose of garbage. On that, no one could disagree. The consul issued a statement urging people to clean up their homes and businesses. But autopsies and diagnoses were different.

City and federal doctors ordered that any Chinese person who died unattended by a physician, or whose medical history was unknown, be autopsied in order to ascertain the cause of death. But autopsies outraged the sensibilities of grieving families and friends. To placate authorities, Ho Yow advised his constituents that, when sick, they should send for a "white physician." If they were too poor to pay, a doctor would be furnished free from the new Oriental Dispensary.

Without an autopsy, however, cases of plague might be mistaken for something else. Plague in the lungs might be misdiagnosed as common pneumonia, fretted city physician O'Brien, who attended to Wong Chut King. The victim suffocates so quickly that the telltale buboes don't have time to erupt, he said. So the city board of health passed a motion ordering that any Chinese dying of apparent pneumonia, swollen glands, fever, or other symptoms of possible plague be subject to autopsy—"the same as whites."[15]

Days after the order was issued, monthly death reports in Chinatown began to *subside*. The mortality rate was half of normal.

Cases of sickness were being concealed, and deaths as well, the health board concluded. One patient who lived across from the Chinese consulate vanished before inspectors arrived. In another case, a man said to have died the day before was as ripe as a week-old corpse. Whether the corpse was in a state of rapid decomposition due to plague or had simply been abandoned for several days was hard to know. The elderly doctor in charge, who worked behind a pharmacy on Kearny Street, denied concealing plague deaths but admitted he was under pressure to dissemble.

Dr. Edward Seltzer recounted to the health board his hellish house call. He found the patient "unable to lie down, and unable to sit up, and was doubled over suffering terribly, spitting blood and suffocating. . . . Nothing I could do was of more than at most transient effect, and the man died in my presence. . . . I was a little undecided as to the cause of death, but gave it as lobar pneumonia because the Chinese have a horror of dissection and begged me to give as the cause of death something which could call for no dissection."[16]

Bodies were whisked room to room, stashed in out-of-the-way cubbyholes, or carried over the rooftops—in a shell game to keep the sick and dying from the inspectors. In other cases, San Francisco Bay became a river Styx, with bodies stowed aboard tiny fishing boats, slipped across the water, and interred in an unknown spot. Hiding the dead was Chinatown's defense against the intrusion of white doctors. How many bodies disappeared, no one knew.[17]

Some hid in plain sight. One ingenious ruse involved a game of dominoes. During an inspection on Waverly Place in Chinatown, one doctor found five men seated around a game table. The players froze as police officers stormed the apartment, upending the place but finding nothing. Two hours later, one of the players was found to be dead. During the inspection, his companions had propped him up at the game table, with his hand poised upon a domino in such a natural position that he escaped notice.

"Their tricks are manifold," said the duped doctor, W. G. Hay of the University of California, in a speech to the California Academy of Medicine. Just how to outsmart the inspectors, he fumed, "[t]he wily heathen seemed to know by instinct."[18]

Rants against the "heathen" Chinese made Consul Ho Yow heartsick. His ailing constituents were forced to flee for fear of the rough interventions of the white doctors, he said, but he denied that his people were actually hiding the dead.[19]

An exodus of Chinese began, driven by fears of quarantine, chemical bombardment, and needles. Some scattered to the gardens and factories of their friends in the suburbs. Others were quartered as cooks in private homes within the city. At the old Globe Hotel, the usual three hundred tenants had dwindled to a dozen, who stood with their bags packed, ready to leave if the cordons went up or the torch was threatened again.

On the waterfront, Dr. Kinyoun tried to assert his authority as quarantine officer. But his bluster failed to hold back a rising tide of derision. When a steamer called the *Gaelic* arrived from Asia with a sick Chinese man aboard, Kinyoun quarantined the vessel. Somehow, despite Kinyoun's ban on reporters in quarantine, one from the *Examiner* managed to sneak aboard or to smuggle out stories of Kinyoun in action. The paper published an account of Kinyoun charging about the deck, barking orders, behaving as a bully, acting overbearing to the poor and obsequious to the rich.[20]

The city board of health, meanwhile, had no cash to pay for the cleanup. The health board begged the board of supervisors for $7,500 to pay men to fork garbage into the incinerator, to sprinkle formaldehyde and shovel lime about Chinatown. The bid for funds inflamed suspicions that the plague was merely a pretext for padding the budget. Newspaper cartoons showed Kinyoun's monkey, rat, and guinea pig as burglars robbing the city treasury. The *Chung Sai Yat Po* declared: "If the government didn't have this $7,500 Buddha, nobody could frame us with the plague."[21]

News of San Francisco's misfortune became impossible to contain, and dispatches reached other states and countries both north and south of the border. Westbound trains traveled empty, abandoned by those afraid of contracting the deadly bacteria. Vacationers favored safer destinations where the greatest concern was sunburn or overeating.

Trading partners began to balk at receiving the city's infected goods. The Canadian government ordered all steamers from San Francisco quarantined until further notice. And the outbound steamer *Curaçao* was quarantined in Mazatlán by the government of Mexico. San Francisco businessmen remembered how quarantine had paralyzed Hawaiian sugar shipments after Honolulu's plague struck. A sickening vision of California wheat stranded on the docks, and its fruit rotting, rose before their eyes.

Editorial pages of the city's major dailies called it an outrage that the city was being branded a pestilential plague spot rather than the golden vision of health and pleasure they wanted to promote.

Down at the intersection of Market and Kearny—the Times Square of the West—publishers displayed their edifice complex. The de Young family erected the West's first steel-frame skyscraper for the *Chronicle*'s headquarters, rising a majestic ten stories. Then William Randolph Hearst hired the same architects to design a loftier tower for the *Examiner* just across the street. He was topped by Claus Spreckels, the sugar king, who built his newspaper, the *Call,* a nineteen-story monument.[22]

Although rivals in every other respect, de Young's *Chronicle* and Spreckels's *Call* found themselves on the same side of an issue. Both papers relentlessly ridiculed the plague campaign of Kinyoun as a fraud. Ironically, the only newspaper of the big three dailies to engage in serious coverage of the outbreak was that font of yellow journalism, Hearst's *Examiner.* To be sure, the so-called saffron sheet pursued the plague story less for its public health import than for its sensational ingredients of death and intrigue. But in the city, its coverage stood alone. Now, however, other city papers charged the *Examiner* with journalistic treason against San Francisco. Hearst's *New York Journal* spread news of the city's shame, declaring: BLACK PLAGUE CREEPS INTO AMERICA.[23]

In a stunning admission on March 25, the *Call*'s editors admitted that they and the *Chronicle*'s editors had made a mutual pact of silence on the plague. They blasted the *Examiner* for its heresy. "It will be remembered that the *Call* and the *Chronicle* agreed to omit publication of the sensational doings of the Board of Health and the Chief of Police . . . but the *Examiner* not only refused to join this proper policy, but wired the lying report to the *New York Journal* and thence spread it broadcast."

As the rhetoric mounted, furious merchants converged on City Hall. They vowed the yellow flag of plague would never fly over San Francisco and demanded that the mayor repair the damage to the city's image.

Mayor Phelan had no choice. He dispatched telegrams to forty American cities, insisting—falsely—that there had been just one isolated case, adding that Chinatown was purged and purified. "There is no future danger," he promised.

Over the page one story, the *Call* unfurled a banner headline: CITY PLAGUE SCARE A CONFESSED SHAM.[24]

As City Hall capitulated to the merchants and newspapers, Kinyoun confirmed three new plague deaths. Word by word, the public health service expanded its codebook. In it, San Francisco's beleaguered health board acquired a code name that captured the style of the whole town—"Burlesque."

A New Quarantine

YELLOW SULFUR FUMES CAST an amber pall over Chinatown. The Chinese choked and cursed the caustic fog. But the health department insisted the haze was a sign of progress against the plague.

Lim Fa Muey, a teenage cigar maker, was one of those who hurried to work through the veil of chemicals one morning in early May 1900. Once she was inside the cigar factory, the familiar tang of cured tobacco leaves would have been welcome after the stench of fumigation—if it weren't that she began to feel so ill. The same symptoms that hit her neighbors now assailed the girl. They were the symptoms of a disease that officially didn't exist: the leaden ache that dragged at her back and limbs. The lurching stomach. The giddy head. The eyes that burned fever bright.

Back at her apartment at 739 Clay Street that evening, her body ached like an old woman's. Inside, the bacteria overflowed from her lymph glands into her bloodstream, invading tissues of her heart, liver, and spleen. The germ's poison dissolved vessel walls, so that the blood seeped out in small hemorrhages that bloomed like ink stains beneath the skin. As her cells lost the battle against the invader, the rising fever burned her senseless. From delirium, she lapsed into coma. Her pulse sped, then sank to an imperceptible flutter. One by one, her organs failed. Her heart stopped. On May 11, Lim Fa Muey became the city's first female plague victim, but not the last.[1]

On the same day, Minnie Worley, a white physician working in

Chinatown, made a house call at 730½ Commercial Street. A family had called her to examine their teenage maid, Chin Moon. While cleaning house, Chin Moon felt a sudden wave of dizziness. She tried to continue her chores, but the vertigo forced her to lie down. Now her head throbbed. She ached from her skull to the pit of her stomach. She vomited and felt better, but only briefly. The pain was relentless. Her lower right abdomen was tender, and she winced at the doctor's touch. Her temperature was 105 degrees Fahrenheit. Her pulse raced at 120 beats per minute.[2]

Dr. Worley diagnosed typhoid fever. It was a safe guess, in a day when the typhoid germ lived in tainted milk and water, but Worley was wrong. By morning, Chin Moon was delirious. Sinking into a coma, the unresponsive girl was taken by carriage to Pacific Hospital, but the doctors there were helpless to save her. In the predawn dark of Sunday morning, May 13, she died.

Drs. Kinyoun and Kellogg brought the body of Chin Moon back to the Chinese hospital for an autopsy. There, they discovered the one crucial symptom that Dr. Worley had overlooked: a lump on the inside of the girl's right thigh. They lanced the lump and exposed a skein of inflamed lymph glands. After drawing fluid into a syringe, they squirted it onto a glass slide and looked at it through the microscope. They saw short, rounded, rod-shaped bacteria. When stained by Gram's method, the germs glowed with the pink hue of plague.

Unmoved by these findings, Dr. Worley stood by her diagnosis of typhoid. Chin Moon's killer couldn't have been plague, she argued. Nobody in her employer's household—including four women, four children, and several men—had caught the disease from her.[3] She didn't understand that though typhoid races from person to person, via unclean hands, food, and water, plague usually needs a middleman to spread it. The city had no idea that plague most often is spread not by people, but by the capricious appetite of a rat flea.

By mid-May, nine people had officially died from the plague. As he wired Washington about each new case of "bumpkin," Kinyoun was worried. The local health board, while calling for antiplague measures to stop the outbreak, had limited funds and no experience in epidemic control. Worse, it seemed impossible to extract a medical history from the Chinese.

Terrified of having their homes or shops invaded, the Chinese volunteered little. When asked about a sick or dead relative or neighbor, people often said the deceased had been ill for a month. A long-drawn-out death was at odds with the short, violent course of the plague. Kinyoun suspected that those interviewed were coached to conceal the plague. He felt like a fool, intentionally misled, but he was helpless to stop it.

Surgeon General Wyman resorted to diplomatic maneuvers. He sent a strongly worded letter to Wu Ting-Fang, China's envoy in Washington, D.C.: "I would respectfully suggest that you send a dispatch to your Consul-General in San Francisco . . . to use his influence to have the Chinese comply cheerfully with necessary measures of the health officials, and to confer with Surgeon Kinyoun, Angel Island. . . ."[4]

In a May 15 telegram to Kinyoun, Surgeon General Wyman outlined a master plan for plague control: "Cordon [off] suspected area; guard ferries and R.R. stations with reference to Chinese only; house to house inspection with Haffkine inoculation; Chinatown to be restricted; pest house in Chinatown . . . ; suspects from plague houses to be moved [if] you deem necessary to Angel Island; a disinfecting corps; destruction of rats. . . ."[5]

This last point—"destruction of rats"—got little immediate attention in the spring of 1900. Wyman had recognized mounting evidence that rats were the chief agents in the spread of plague from port to port, but he hadn't yet seen their connection with the infection of people. A report from Sydney, Australia, where doctors discovered plague bacteria in the stomachs of fleas, received scant notice. Only years later would medical science recognize the significance of these fragmentary bits of evidence implicating the rat and the flea.[6]

The surgeon general also ordered Kinyoun to meet with Consul Ho Yow, to appeal for cooperation. Kinyoun boarded a ferry to San Francisco for an audience with the consul. Ushered in to see Ho Yow, Kinyoun took the measure of the subtle diplomat. He was handsome, clad in the robes of an imperial envoy from the Manchu dynasty. He spoke fluent English.

The city was a hostile territory for those of Chinese descent. When young men of Chinatown offered to join the army of their adopted land, the local press mocked their offer with cartoons of pig-tailed enlistees. When elders shipped their bones home for burial in

China, they were hit with a ten-dollar bone tax. Now came these draconian plague-control measures and an order from the U.S. government to submit "cheerfully." It was too much. Ho insisted on reserving certain basic rights for his people.

Kinyoun had begun to brief Ho on the plague outbreak when a knock on the door brought another visitor. The attorney for the Chinese Six Companies entered. Two against one. Ho and the attorney made their case: The Chinese people were terrified of the needle. They would not submit to forced vaccination. They would not stand for forced relocation to detention centers here or on Angel Island.

Kinyoun felt ambushed, outgunned. Up to this point, he had thought of the Chinese Six Companies mainly as a trade association to protect rich merchants' interests, but now he saw that they functioned as de facto diplomats. Tough negotiators, they would not have public health forced upon them. "Just there, I believe, the opposition to the Marine-Hospital Service, and particularly myself, originated," he told a friend.[7] Far from eliciting the cheerful compliance Wyman envisioned, Kinyoun made no allies that day.

On the streets of Chinatown, and in its press, Kinyoun was dubbed "wolf doctor," for what they perceived as his snappy and officious manner toward the Chinese.[8] If Kinyoun was the wolf doctor, the Chinese refused to be his sacrificial lambs. Most people knew the story of the Haffkine vaccine and its risks: fever, weakness, and even death. From his window at the consular residence, Ho Yow saw angry crowds gathering in the streets. He wired his minister in Washington to seek to cancel the compulsory vaccine order. "The Chinese . . . would prefer to be kicked back to China. They are very upset and agitated. We are afraid that a riot might happen and that people might be killed. Please go to the Federal Government and plead for an exemption from the shots."[9]

Word spread about the little girl at the Presbyterian Mission Home who leapt out a window to evade the white men's needles, her shattered bones an emblem of the community's broken trust.[10] Demonstrators swarmed like angry bees from a hive, the *Chung Sai Yat Po* reported.[11] Chinatown merchants declared a one-day strike, closing their shops in protest against the immunization order. Along the bustling bazaar of Dupont Street, sales of housewares, silks, and ceramics ceased. The street was still and shuttered.

If anything, the rebellion only stiffened the resolve of Surgeon General Wyman to force the Chinese into compliance. Invoking the Quarantine Act of 1890, Wyman was authorized by President William McKinley to issue a sweeping order—not just halting travel by plague patients, but forbidding train or boat travel by all "Asiatics and other races particularly liable to the disease." Now, railroad and shipping companies refused to sell tickets to Asian passengers. No Asian could leave the state without a health certificate issued by Kinyoun. And that required the dreaded Haffkine vaccine.[12]

It was Kinyoun's job to enforce the order. The travel ban covered both Chinese and Japanese people. Clusters of Japanese lived and worked near the borders of Chinatown, but as yet no single case of plague had been found in a Japanese resident of San Francisco. It was a clear case of quarantine by color.

Challenges to the ban came quickly. After merchants like Louis Quong were barred from boarding the Oakland ferry, a class-action lawsuit was filed in federal court. Wong Wai, a businessman associated with the Chinese Six Companies, filed the suit charging Kinyoun and the board of health with illegally imprisoning twenty-five thousand Chinese inside San Francisco unless they took the experimental and dangerous Haffkine vaccine.[13] The lawsuit charged that the travel restrictions were unconstitutional and demanded that Kinyoun and the health board be enjoined from requiring vaccination or barring their travel.

Left to untangle the snarl of competing federal and local health and civil rights claims was Judge William W. Morrow. Before he ascended the bench, the silver-haired jurist had been a three-term Republican member of Congress. As a lawmaker, Morrow wasn't known for his love of the Chinese, whom he once labeled "destitute of moral qualities." As a judge hearing exclusion-law cases, he often sided with the government.[14]

But on May 28, Judge Morrow ruled in favor of the Chinese. The defendants, Joseph Kinyoun and the city health board, failed to furnish facts that justified singling out the city's Asian residents as more susceptible to plague. The travel restrictions and forced immunization weren't dictated by sound science, but instead were "boldly directed against the Asiatic or Mongolian race as a class, without regard to the previous condition, habits, exposure to the disease or residence of the individual; and the only justification offered for this discrimination was a suggestion [that] this particular race is more liable to plague than any other," the judge wrote. "No evidence has, however, been offered to support this claim. . . ."[15]

In his decision in the Wong Wai case, Judge Morrow also ruled that ordering the city's twenty-five thousand Chinese residents to take the Haffkine vaccine as a condition of travel violated Surgeon General Wyman's own medical judgment. The vaccine was good only before exposure to the germ, not afterward. Giving the vaccine to someone after exposure was not only ineffective, but indeed "dangerous to life." Giving it to people leaving an infected zone served no public health aim. Thus the whole program—travel restrictions and vaccine—discriminated against Chinese residents, depriving them of liberty in violation of the equal protection clause of the Fourteenth Amendment of the Constitution. Judge Morrow issued an injunction.

Kinyoun and the city health board, the judge added, failed to prove that there was a plague emergency serious enough to warrant the suspension of rights and due process. The injunction was to remain in effect while the case was being litigated. Word of the plague in San Francisco was seeping out. Texas and Louisiana declared an embargo against all California passengers and goods. And now, the only plan for curbing the infection was halted by court order.

As negative publicity mounted, the California State Health Board jumped into the fray. In a surprise move, it ordered the city to restore the quarantine and threatened to quarantine the entire city from the rest of the state of California if it did not comply. The state board wasn't admitting the existence of plague—far from it; it was just trying to limit the damage from negative publicity, and shield California's trade and tourism from a devastating embargo.

In a meeting at the Grand Hotel, the state health board invited local businesspeople to meet with the Southern Pacific Railroad Company and the Fruit Canners' Union. The fractious crowd was split as to whether quarantine was a necessary evil or a devastating admission to the world that California crops were tainted. Debate was loud and furious.

Dr. Williamson of the San Francisco Health Board despaired that his hands were tied. The local press and businesses billed the plague cleanup as a fraud, and the court injunction left him hamstrung.

But D. D. Crowley of the California State Health Board was unmoved. Crowley had his own preference, and that was to burn Chinatown to the ground. But if he couldn't use the torch, a fence would do. "Gentlemen," he ordered at the close of the May 28 meeting, "you must have Chinatown quarantined this evening."[16] With Sacramento holding a gun to its head, the San Francisco Board of Supervisors passed a resolution empowering the health board to quarantine Chinatown for a second time.

Once again, 159 police officers descended on Chinatown. They guarded the district twenty-four hours a day in three shifts, sealing off the rectangle bounded by Stockton, Kearny, California, and Broadway. Now the quarantine zone was enlarged by one block to the north. But again, it zigzagged to exempt white institutions, including the redbrick steeple of St. Mary's Church at California and Dupont Streets.

Chinatown churned in helpless frustration as the normal ebb and flow of business between whites and Asians was interrupted. A white woman on Stockton tried to pass garments to a Chinese tailor, but a police officer blocked the exchange. A Chinese man tried to mail a letter outside the zone, but guards spun him around and hustled him back to his quarter. A laundryman staggered up to the rope line under a heap of clean clothes for delivery outside the zone. An officer halted the shipment.[17]

The first time, it was a penetrable quarantine made of flimsy ropes, but this time, the barricades were hardened with wooden fence posts and barbed wire. A persistent buzz in the neighborhood said the quarantine was a mere prelude to imprisonment. Wyman and Kinyoun were exchanging telegrams discussing a proposal for the mass relocation of the Chinese to plague detention camps on Angel Island near the quarantine station, or on Mission Rock, a tiny, desolate speck of land in the bay near the waterfront warehouses. The news shot a new bolt of fear through the Chinese. Detention camps were a throwback to the medieval lazarettos, isolation hospitals or pesthouses.

Back East, wire service stories about San Francisco's plague cases were now seeping into the press. With a major news event brewing out West, the dean of New York medical reporters decided to investigate. Dr. George F. Shrady, the burly, bearded medical correspondent for the *New York Herald,* boarded a train west to determine once and for all whether bubonic plague really existed in San Francisco.

The surgeon general got wind of the reporting trip. Fretting about bad publicity, he commanded Kinyoun to call upon the influential journalist at his hotel and brief him on the plague situation.

Kinyoun fumed. It was like bringing the mountain to Mohammed. Choking back his resentment, he boarded a ferry to the city. From the Ferry Building, he rode west on Market Street to the Palace Hotel on New Montgomery. He walked through the cobblestoned coaches' entrance, under seven stories of balconies and a glass atrium roof. Once past the 150-foot dining room ablaze with chandeliers, he caught an elevator to Dr. Shrady's room. The Palace's rooms had fifteen-foot ceilings, bay windows, coffee served on Haviland china from France, and beds of imported Irish linen. It was the hostelry he could not afford, the scene of his first humiliation by this city, and now the scene of his second.

"I called upon the Doctor and after much struggling I was admitted to the presence," Kinyoun told a friend. "I found him stowed away up in the Palace, surrounded by stenographers, typewriters, confidential clerks, bell boys, and porters, running as it were, the whole editorial business of the *Herald.*"[18]

Shrady assured Kinyoun that he had the editorial freedom to print the truth in his paper, adding that the *Call* would syndicate his series. Kinyoun suspected that Shrady's real agenda was to deny plague had existed before his arrival and then to "discover" it during his stay and plant the *Herald*'s flag on the story. It was an old reporter's trick, that of reinventing the news. But Kinyoun duly briefed Shrady on the plague cases diagnosed so far and invited him to view an autopsy. As it happened, the plague inconveniently went into hiding that week, so there was little to show.

Shrady toured the plague zone and reported what he saw, but he had to acknowledge that he had yet to see a single living case of plague. However, he reported that Kinyoun showed him all the clinical charts, autopsy notes, and lab tests amassed so far. All this, Shrady said, convinced him that the bubonic plague was real.

"Microscopic preparations . . . [and] infected organs said to have been removed from the nine dead bodies . . . now leave such mute but valuable testimony for accurate scientific investigation," wrote Shrady. "I personally examined every one of them and the existence of bubonic plague bacillus in all of them admits of no shadow of doubt."[19]

With a police escort kicking down doors, Shrady returned to tour Chinatown alcoves by candlelight, hoping to see a live plague patient as evidence of the epidemic. It eluded him.

Still, Shrady planned to write an incendiary finale. "He was going to advocate the total destruction of Chinatown by fire, by destruction by dynamite, drive these people out from their abodes," Kinyoun said. At a time when the vaccine campaign was provoking the Chinese to open revolt, Kinyoun said, "I begged him by everything holy never to advocate such a thing as that at the present time unless he had ten thousand troops at his back."[20]

May 30 was Memorial Day, and the streets were draped in bunting, lined with patriotic crowds waving flags and brass bands blaring martial tunes. Amid the festivities, Kinyoun and Kellogg learned of a new suspicious death in Chinatown. They invited Shrady to attend the postmortem.

After pressing through the cheering parade throngs, the trio of doctors got passes to cross the quarantine line and made their way toward their grim errand. Once they reached the morgue, they had to run a gauntlet of angry and mistrustful Chinese before entering. There, they unwrapped a shroud covering the corpse of a forty-year-old laborer, Dang Hong, dressed in his funeral robes.

"All the pathologic phenomena observed were those usually associated with plague," Shrady wrote. ". . . On the left side under the jaw, there were evidences of suppuration, due to previous inflammation of the glands. . . . The glands in the groin were slightly enlarged. . . . Numerous specimens were removed from the body for future microscopical observation by Drs. Kellogg and Kinyoun." Later, Kellogg came to Shrady's hotel with a specimen for Shrady to examine. Both men agreed: The samples contained the bacteria of bubonic plague.[21]

Indignantly, the *Chung Sai Yat Po* attacked the diagnosis. The paper deemed the autopsy suspicious because the Chinese Six Companies' own observers were barred from attending it. "The Chinese knew very well that he did not die of plague," the Chinese reporter wrote. "They wanted to find out what those wicked doctors were doing." He compared the Caucasian doctors to greedy vultures attacking carrion. "Perhaps there is a ghost of plague haunting Chinatown," he wrote. "To quarantine Chinatown is to eat the meat of the ghost of the plague. Do you think there is enough meat for them?"[22]

After his story on the autopsy of Dang Hong, Shrady became something of a celebrity in San Francisco. The *Call* reprinted his series. Even the Chinese daily ran his story.[23] Kinyoun nursed hopes that this reporter, for all his arrogance, might yet help the plague campaign by writing truthful dispatches. It looked as if that might come to pass. Then, suddenly, Shrady turned from alarmist to apologist.

Shrady's conversion followed a banquet thrown in his honor by Mayor Phelan at the posh Pacific Union Club. Surrounded by city politicians, Shrady tucked into an elaborate procession of courses at a table garlanded with flowers and cornucopias of California fruits. The visiting journalist rode through Golden Gate Park to the Cliff House, to breathe the sea air while overlooking the Pacific surf. Before retiring for the night at the Palace, Shrady told the press he was charmed by the city's pleasures. Later that night, who should drop by Shrady's hotel for a chat but California's governor, Henry T. Gage.[24]

"The dinner had the desired effect," Kinyoun later wrote to his family in the East. "The Doctor [Shrady] had evidently been doctored."[25]

After being entertained, Shrady published a finale to his plague series, in which he withdrew any concern he'd earlier expressed:

"After having visited every section of Chinatown under the escort of the police and of the health authorities, both Federal and local, I have come to the conclusion that this plague scare in San Francisco is absolutely unwarranted," Shrady wrote. "I am thoroughly convinced that there really was no danger of the plague and that virtually it did not exist in this city."

"The rumor that plague threatens San Francisco is ridiculous and unfounded," he concluded. "One swallow does not make a summer, and one case of plague does not make an epidemic."[26]

Kinyoun was crushed. Now, he feared, the East Coast would never learn the truth from Shrady. "The Philistines," he said, "had shorn him of his locks."[27]

On the same day that the newspaperman recanted, Chew Kuey

Kem, a forty-nine-year-old cigar maker, died in Chinatown—one more case of "bumpkin" for the books.

With the city's trade and prestige at stake, the *Call* pleaded "in the name of humanity" for Chinatown to be burned. "So long as it stands, so long will there be the menace of the appearence in San Francisco of every form of disease, plague and pestilence which Asian filth and vice generate," the paper said in its May 31 editorial. "Clear the foul spot from San Francisco and give its debris to the flames."

The Wolf Doctor

◉

PLAGUE CASES NOW HOPSCOTCHED randomly across Chinatown. As doctors puzzled over the elusive link among the dozen people who had died, they began marking cases on the map of Chinatown
with pastel-colored pencil dots—pale green for 1900. Later, they
would switch to marking red dots and black crosses for each case of
sickness or death. The dots on the map multiplied.

But as the second quarantine stretched on, hunger afflicted the
residents of Chinatown more than the plague did. There was nothing
to buy and no money to buy it. The Chinese Six Companies asked the
city for 25 cents a day to feed the hungry. But a city health board
member vetoed the request as too high; the almshouse, he said, fed
its inmates for 8 cents a day.[1]

The city made a strategic counteroffer, dangling food relief as an
incentive to the Chinese to move to the detention centers being
planned for Mission Rock or Angel Island. The Chinese Six Companies refused: It was better to be hungry and free than fed in prison.
The Chinese vowed to resist relocation by law or by force.

The desperation of the Chinese was scarcely noticed by most
whites. And when it was, as it was by a story in the *Call* on June 3, it
was spiked with sarcasm:

CHINESE ENDS LIFE IN A
NOVEL MANNER

Le Chow, a Chinese confined within the quarantined district, became tired of life and chose a novel means of escaping from this vale of tears. He broke the bulb of a thermometer and swallowed the mercury. In a short time, his troubles were over and the Board of Health now has his body for autopsy.

While the newspapers turned a suicide into slapstick, a few Chinese took their anger to court. Jew Ho, a grocer on Stockton Street, was incensed to discover that the cordons encircling his store curved to exclude a white plumber and coal dealer next door. Starved of business, he filed a lawsuit on June 5, charging that the quarantine violated his constitutional guarantee of equal protection under the law. He demanded that Caucasian physicians not be barred from crossing the quarantine line to attend their Chinese patients.[2]

Like other lawsuits before it, the heart of Jew Ho's claim was that there was no plague in San Francisco. But even if there were plague, the suit argued, a mass quarantine didn't protect the Chinese but heightened their risk by sealing them up inside an infected district. The complaint asked the court to end the quarantine and restrict isolation to only the infected homes and shops.

Kinyoun backed the city's plan to round up the Chinese and relocate them to Angel Island or Mission Rock. But the circuit court issued a temporary restraining order barring Chinese detention centers. The court allowed doctors designated by the Chinese Six Companies to cross the quarantine lines to see their patients.[3]

Criminals hungrily exploited the situation. There was a brisk trade in counterfeit health certificates. And a Caucasian man—never identified—falsely promised to raise the quarantine for $10,000. Chinese merchants began raising the cash. Newspapers exposed the fraud, but the con man was never caught.[4]

Agitated Chinese—one thousand strong—descended on Portsmouth Square, where quarantine officers had pitched tents to give shots and fumigate clothing of people who had to cross the quarantine lines. Rumors were circulating that the officers were forcibly inoculating the Chinese with the Haffkine vaccine. Special police—

detailed to keep peace inside the quarantine lines—charged at the crowds, brandishing their clubs and dispersing the demonstrators. But the mob ran uphill and assembled at a shop on Waverly Place, where the owner was believed to be collaborating with the white doctors. This time, the police lines couldn't hold them back.

Hurling cobblestones pried from the street, the Chinese demonstrators smashed the shop windows and then charged into the shop, breaking up furniture and pitching pieces onto the sidewalk. The next day, as the shopkeeper surveyed the ruins of his store, the newspapers reported that there was no forced vaccination plot. The Chinese who entered the tents that day did so willingly, so they could have their clothes fumigated and leave Chinatown to join a shipping expedition to Siberia.[5]

A delivery to a Chinatown coffin shop was the spark that ignited a second riot. Seething crowds saw the approach of the lumbering delivery wagon and believed the coffin shipment was part of a plot to make it look as if a rampant epidemic were under way. As the horse cart entered Chinatown, swaying under its somber freight, three hundred demonstrators attacked it, dumping empty coffins onto the cobblestones of Sacramento Street. Then they ransacked the coffin shop, tearing down hangings and heaving furniture into the street.

Uniformed officers struck savagely with their clubs, raining blows on the demonstrators. "Heads were not spared," the *Call* commented. "The police were unusually severe but the case demanded it. Rioting . . . cannot be permitted."[6]

In court, the Chinese relentlessly pounded away at the theme that the quarantine was an act of racial bias, not public health. "Real prison has iron bars," said the counsel for the Chinese Six Companies, a former judge named James Maguire. "But when you surround the area with ropes and hurdles and restrict the freedom of the people, it is also imprisonment," he said. "Do they want to starve 10,000 Chinese to death?"[7] Now the Chinese launched a private food drive, distributing rations of rice, cabbage, and pork.

Judge John J. De Haven chiseled the first legal chip off the quarantine by granting a habeas corpus petition. He ordered the release of a Chinese cook who lived with his white employers on Bush Street but who got trapped in the quarantine zone while visiting friends in Chinatown. Judge De Haven forbade the health board from restricting the liberty of anyone—Asian or white—who wasn't in direct contact with the plague.[8]

In Washington, the Chinese minister Wu Ting-Fang sent the U.S. government a bill for $30,000 for each day his subjects were incarcerated in Chinatown. Presented with this bill, Secretary of State John Hay wired Governor Gage, asking whether plague really existed in California.

On June 14, Governor Gage issued a fourteen-point proclamation denying that there was any plague in "the great and healthful city of San Francisco."

Gage's no-plague manifesto bore the signatures of San Francisco's elite, including blue jeans manufacturer Levi Strauss. Plague was, after all, bad for business. But in a shocking show of complicity, the deans of three medical schools also signed the denial, including Levi Cooper Lane, president of Cooper Medical College, which would become Stanford University Medical School. None had firsthand experience with bubonic plague.[9]

On June 15, the courtroom was packed to hear arguments in the Jew Ho lawsuit. Consul Ho Yow was there, as were forty Christian missionaries and about a hundred Chinese spectators. Ng Poon Chew, the crusading editor of the *Chung Sai Yat Po,* took furious notes.

Jew Ho called a parade of expert medical witnesses, who gave sworn testimony that there was no plague. Physician Minnie Worley asserted that the young maid Chin Moon had died of typhoid fever. Judge Morrow listened attentively from the bench. If it were the court's job to rule on the truth of the diagnosis, Judge Morrow said, "I think upon such testimony as that given by these physicians I should be compelled to hold that the plague did not exist and has not existed in San Francisco."[10]

Though it wasn't the court's job to settle matters of science, Judge Morrow threw the quarantine out on legal grounds. It lumped all Chinese homes and businesses together, while exempting white-occupied buildings. It didn't distinguish between homes of plague-infected and homes of healthy Chinese, but confined them all together, increasing risk of transmission. It forbade the Chinese from access to physicians of their choice. For all these reasons, said Judge Morrow, echoing the U.S. Supreme Court in a prior discrimination case, the San Francisco quarantine was imposed with "an evil eye and an unequal hand."

"This quarantine," he went on, "cannot be continued by reason of the fact that it is unreasonable, unjust, and oppressive . . . discriminating in its character [and] contrary to the provisions of the Fourteenth Amendment of the Constitution of the United States."[11]

Within hours of Judge Morrow's ruling, the city health board repealed the quarantine. The good news crackled through the alleyways of Chinatown like a string of New Year firecrackers. Expectant crowds sifted into the streets, swelling and pressing against the barriers near Portsmouth Square. That afternoon, a police wagon pulled up to the intersection of Kearny and Clay. A captain in civilian clothes jumped out, broke down the fences, and rolled up the barbed wire.[12]

Chinese poured through the lines, their lean faces awash with joy and relief. For the first time in two weeks, workers returned to their jobs—shelves were restocked, tables set, and hollow bellies filled.

During the litigation, however, the plague bacteria hadn't slept. New victims fell sick just doors away from the celebration. Containing the plague was like trying to catch quicksilver. Stung by his legal setback and alarmed by the new cases, Kinyoun devised another scheme.

If he couldn't quarantine Chinatown, he would broaden the surgeon general's May 21 prohibition on Asian travel into a sweeping ban on people of any race leaving San Francisco for other places. Ships and trains were ordered to deny tickets to any person without a health certificate signed by Kinyoun. He dashed off urgent letters on June 15 to the Southern Pacific Railroad and the Pacific Coast Steamship Company.[13] With a rising sense of panic, he urged the surgeon general to build detention camps to hold plague suspects at the state border, using War Department tents. "Rush answer," he implored.[14]

Kinyoun also fired off warning letters to the health boards of Louisiana, Texas, Kansas, Nevada, Oregon, Colorado, Arizona, New Mexico, and Washington, urging that they stay on the lookout for any infected passengers or freight from the Golden State.[15]

The explosion was predictable. California's commercial and political powers erupted in fury: At stake was a bumper crop of California fruit worth $40 million and fortunes in transportation and tourism revenues—all paralyzed by Kinyoun's sweeping new decree. Their wrath echoed in a banner headline in the *Call* on June 17, 1900:

CALIFORNIA IS SUBJECTED
TO AN UNPARALLELED
OUTRAGE:
DR. J. J. KINYOUN STRIKES A
SERIOUS BLOW TO THE STATE
BY ARBITRARILY AND WITHOUT
CAUSE PLACING IT UNDER
FEDERAL QUARANTINE.

"The indignation of the people of California is beyond expression," said the Republican State Central Committee.[16] A delegation led by the *Call*'s publisher, John D. Spreckels, took the protest to the door of the White House.

President McKinley didn't take long to overrule Kinyoun's travel ban. Vindicated San Franciscans rejoiced, viewing the president's act as not just a green light for travel, but a clean bill of health for the city.

In the wake of the president's order, Kinyoun was charged with contempt of court. But the governor had an even more nefarious, more effective plan to bury the quarrelsome quarantine officer for good. Gage unveiled a conspiracy theory that would discredit Kinyoun, while offering a convenient way to explain the existence of plague bacteria in his state.

Gage told the press that Kinyoun had imported cultures of bubonic plague bacteria for use in his laboratory on Angel Island, then suggested that, by spilling the bacteria, Kinyoun had created the catastrophe himself.[17]

Kinyoun, captain of a sinking ship, was summoned to court for a hearing before Judge Morrow on the contempt charge. By turns meek and belligerent, Kinyoun gave assurances that he hadn't intended to violate any court order. The *Call* called Kinyoun "insolent and dangerous" and an "injudicious meddler" in state affairs.[18]

Kinyoun got cold comfort from his government-appointed attorney, Frank Coombs, who told the quarantine officer he was going to have a hard time keeping him out of jail.[19]

Judge Morrow gave Kinyoun a week to show cause why he should not be held in contempt of court in violating the injunction handed down by the court in the Wong Wai lawsuit.

On Monday, June 25, the courtoom was packed with business-men and members of the Chinese community. Kinyoun was called to the stand and sworn in. J. C. Campbell, an attorney for the Chinese Six Companies, interrogated him about the racial motives for his plague control.

Prickly and defensive, Kinyoun wrangled with Campbell from the witness box, insisting that he was innocent of discriminatory intent and that his earlier action and the new travel ban were "entirely sepa-rate and distinct."[20] Few in the crowd were moved by his argument.

Just as Kinyoun was trying to convince the court in San Francisco about the plague, Rupert Blue was trying to do much the same thing—convince Washington about the plague outbreak in the Medi-terranean. On June 26, Blue had picked up a copy of the Italian paper *Il Caffaro* and was electrified by the news of plague outbreaks in Xanti, Greece, and Smyrna, Turkey. Previously, the U.S. Public Health reports had published an account of only one such case. Blue updated his superiors about a dozen new plague cases and three deaths. He predicted a major plague invasion of continental Europe from the south.[21] His instinct was right; he was just a continent off target. The real plague invasion was under way in San Francisco—Blue's next assignment.

Kinyoun's court grilling ended on July 2. Judge Morrow promised to render his decision on the contempt charge the next day. Kinyoun's prospects looked dire. As the rest of San Francisco bought sparklers and rockets for a July 4th holiday, the Kinyouns despaired in their cot-tage on Angel Island. Kinyoun encouraged his children to think of his trial as a biblical battle between the forces of good and evil—science and commercialism. His son Conrad declared California to be a land of false prophets where people worshiped the dollar.

"Judge Morrow don't seem to know who my papa is," Conrad said. "Judge Morrow thinks he's the biggest man in the world, but right there he's mistaken, he don't know my papa like I do." With none left to champion him, Kinyoun clung to the boy's defense like a life raft.[22]

On July 3, the quarantine officer, flanked by bail bondsmen, re-turned to court to learn his fate. His opponents were confident. But when Judge Morrow took his place on the bench, he delivered a sur-prise reprive: Kinyoun's travel ban—because it was general and not racially focused—hadn't violated the court's ruling against unlawful imprisonment. In any event, the ban was rendered moot by President McKinley's order. Now Kinyoun was cleared of contempt charges. Stunned, he walked out of court a free man. Free, but despised. On Independence Day, news of his freedom was buried in the newspapers' back pages, among reports of shipwrecks.[23]

Kinyoun hoped to consult Judge Morrow on matters of public health but never managed to catch him at his office. He left his card. One night, he was startled to see the white-haired jurist join him in line for the Angel Island ferry.

Kinyoun and the judge sat down together in the cabin of the ferry as it churned north. Amid a crowd of bay commuters, the two men huddled from the San Francisco waterfront to the shores of Tiburon.

Judge Morrow lectured Kinyoun on the line between federal and state control of public health. Kinyoun, in turn, schooled the judge about the dangers of plague. The judge was impressed enough to ask Kinyoun to help him obtain a new kind of rat poison. As the ferry docked, Kinyoun exulted that he'd made the judge see the light.[24]

But Kinyoun's détente with the judge failed to soften the city's antipathy. Calls grew louder for Kinyoun to leave town. In City Hall, the board of supervisors considered a motion to fire the city board of health, his last scientific allies.

OUST THE FAKERS, demanded the *Call*'s editorial page. "On all grounds, the board and Kinyoun should step down."[25]

White Men's Funerals

UNTIL AUGUST 1900, the plague had claimed only Chinese victims. A rough-hewn teamster named William Murphy would change all that.

By day Murphy drove a horse carriage, making deliveries in Chinatown. At night he put down his reins and picked up an opium pipe, escaping from his daily rut of mud and manure into a vaporous dreamscape.

One day, he felt a rush of fever. His head pounded and his body hurt as though he'd been beaten in a bar brawl. He sweated and shivered convulsively, his thirty-four-year-old drayman's frame now weak as a babe's.

Light-headed and woozy, he dragged himself from his Dupont Street apartment to the City and County Hospital at 26th and Potrero Streets. The doctors made puzzled stabs at a diagnosis. On August 11, William Murphy died. An autopsy revealed him to be the city's first white victim of bubonic plague.[1]

Joseph Kinyoun studied the specimens with a grim vindication. "It is the most beautiful case of plague infection (if such things can be called beautiful) that I have encountered in this epidemic," he said.[2] Murphy's death expanded the outbreak beyond people of Asian blood, but it was Anne Roede's that transcended the boundaries of Chinatown.

Anne Roede, a white nurse, was called to Pacific Avenue to tend a teenage boy suffering from stomach pains and respiratory distress. It was a presumed case of diphtheria. As Nurse Roede bent over his bedside, the boy was seized with nausea. Too quick for her to dodge, he heaved and spattered the nurse's face. She cleaned her patient, then composed herself as best she could.

Forty-eight hours later, Nurse Roede felt her own face grow flushed, her throat thick and raw. Her strength swooned, and her breath became labored. Doctors admitted her to the contagious disease ward of Children's Hospital on California Street, another suspected case of diphtheria. Her fever soared. After hovering three days on the fringes of consciousness, the twenty-eight-year-old nurse suffocated.

The doctors moved her body to the Children's Hospital morgue for autopsy and began their postmortem. Only when they looked into her lungs did they realize that Nurse Roede had died of pneumonic plague.

Panic-stricken hospital administrators decided that their morgue was contaminated and that it must be burned. As the fire engines pulled up and prepared to torch the room, someone called for coal oil to drench the floor. The oil was stored in the next room, amid a huge powder keg of flammable fuels—enough to engulf the whole hospital and all of California Street in flames. At the last moment, the fire was canceled. "If it had been started after that manner," Kinyoun reflected, "all the fire engines in San Francisco would not have saved the Children's Hospital."[3]

Nurse Roede's teenage patient died and was buried without an autopsy. Kinyoun was convinced that his killer was pneumonic plague and that he had infected Nurse Roede. He was even more convinced that a chain of such misdiagnoses was concealing the true size of the outbreak. "There have been more cases of bubonic plague . . . in San Francisco than have seen the light," he wrote. "Either deliberately or unintentionally cases of bubonic plague have been returned to the Health Office under another name."[4]

But plague was only part of his job. Quarantine duties had kept him very busy. In just over a year as San Francisco's quarantine officer, Kinyoun had overseen the inspection of more than one thousand ships, during which more than fourteen thousand passengers had been disinfected.[5] Clad in oilskins, the quarantine officers were required to board ships in the bay until nine or ten o'clock at night, breasting the whitecaps, hauling fumigation equipment aboard, smoking and spraying the fetid compartments. They checked passengers and crew, taking temperatures, peering into throats, and palpating glands in the neck to search for any signs of illness aboard ship. Passengers were always restive in quarantine, bridling at the health and baggage checks. It was a wet, grueling, thankless job.

But no ship made waves like the Occidental and Oriental Steam Ship Co. vessel the *Coptic*. She regularly plied the sea lanes from San Francisco through Honolulu and Kobe, Japan, to China, returning with her hold full of China tea, Hawaiian sugarcane, crates of Asian-Pacific delicacies—water chestnuts, yams, green ginger, taro root, lily bulbs, dried fish, and oysters—and a menagerie of dogs, cats, and monkeys.

After leaving San Francisco on June 26, 1900, to return to Asia, the ship's surgeon, James Moloney, documented one of the most contentious cases of an already contentious year. In his ship's logs, the surgeon said the *Coptic* picked up passengers in Honolulu, then headed for Japan. When the ship reached the port of Kobe, a steerage passenger was found mortally ill with fever.[6]

Ah Sow, a twenty-seven-year-old rice farmer from a plantation outside Honolulu, had a temperature of 105 degrees and an egg-size lump erupting from his thigh. Carried ashore in the wee hours, the man died as "the first case of plague occurring in the history of the Pacific Ocean on an outward bound ship," Moloney said.[7]

On the steerage deck near the dead man's berth, inspectors found three dead rats in the scuppers. A frenzy of finger-pointing ensued. The ship's surgeon blamed the passenger Ah Sow for bringing plague aboard the *Coptic* from Hawaii.[8] Honolulu health officers insisted that plague rats already on the ship from San Francisco had infected Ah Sow.

While health officers of California, Hawaii, and the shipping company wrangled, the *Coptic*, now scrubbed and fumigated, raced waves and weather to cross the Pacific again. When she next reached San Francisco Bay, Kinyoun was away, up north inspecting quarantine stations in Canada. He left the San Francisco station in the hands of an experienced officer, who scrutinized the *Coptic*'s freight and passengers to howls of protest over the delay.

Kinyoun returned to San Francisco from Canada to find himself blamed for the *Coptic*'s delayed docking and for alleged rough treatment of the passengers. He wrote to the surgeon general, saying that the unfounded charges were part of a plot to oust him. "I cannot be bribed, coerced or cajoled into a suppression [of the facts] regarding the plague."[9]

By now, Kinyoun's own health was compromised. "I have not been well since I came to San Francisco," he acknowledged to his friends. "I had four break-downs in the last year."[10] His gut, always in turmoil, was seized with pains he ascribed to "chronic appendicitis." Modern doctors might have labeled his malady as ulcers or spastic colon. By any name, there was little relief. In the days before acid blockers and antispasmodic drugs, the public relied on patent medicines laced with alcohol, coca, or morphine. Kinyoun simply suffered and blamed his agony on overwork and political pressure that the *Coptic* affair promised only to exacerbate.

When the *Coptic* next docked in San Francisco on December 14, once again loaded with exotic foodstuffs and live animals Kinyoun suspected were possible carriers of infection, he ordered extraordinary vigilance. He granted limited pratique, meaning only routine cargo could be unloaded, but seafood and produce needed special certificates. Dogs, cats, and monkeys required inspection.[11]

At the wharf, resentment flared as irate merchants sat idly awaiting their shipments. Around the customs house, it was whispered that California's congressmen were lobbying for Kinyoun's transfer "as far away from San Francisco as possible."[12]

San Francisco's Chamber of Commerce president, Charles Nelson, called Kinyoun "a menace to our trade and commerce."[13] On December 21, the Chinese Six Companies sued for release of their goods, charging that Kinyoun had again overreached his authority as quarantine officer.[14]

Now, barely six months free of litigation, Kinyoun was under renewed legal fire. Christmas on Angel Island was somber. Kinyoun took solace in his children's hopes for the holiday. Alice, a pianist, craved music. Perry was obsessed with hunting and fishing. Conrad tickled Kinyoun by having picked up his father's taste for technology and requesting that almost all his presents be machines. "It was real amusing," Kinyoun wrote his friends, "in looking over the list which he gave me for Santa Claus." Otherwise, the holiday held little cheer.[15]

As 1900 drew to a close, the newspapers ran rosy prophecies for San Francisco, now ranked as the nation's eighth largest city, with a population of 342,000. "In San Francisco, the century goes out brilliantly," wrote the *Call's* publisher, John D. Spreckels. "All kinds of trade report a good movement at profitable prices. The export trade of the port was never better . . . the Orient keeps the ships and the shippers busy . . . there is a general feeling of confidence in . . . 1901."[16]

Kinyoun took a gloomier view. "It appears to me that commercial interests of San Francisco are more dear to the inhabitants than the preservation of human life," he wrote. "No sentiment has been expressed against a possible danger arising to the people, to their wives and children. These people seem perfectly indifferent whether or not bubonic plague exists in San Francisco, so long as they can sell their products and make large percentages on their investments."[17]

The *San Francisco Chronicle,* in its year-end editorial, demanded the quarantine officer's expulsion. Headlined THE DOOM OF KINYOUN, the column declared: "Kinyoun is to go. . . . The official acts of Kinyoun have been outrageous, and have fully warranted the public indignation. . . . It is grossly improper for his Federal superiors to say that such a man must not be removed 'under fire.' "[18]

Kinyoun wrote a friend, "I am at war with everybody out here."[19]

In Sacramento, Governor Henry T. Gage escalated his attacks. In his year-end address—a rhetorical volcano that spouted twenty thousand words and covered fifty-four sheets of foolscap—he took his plague conspiracy theory to new and gothic heights. Now instead of just spilling the germs, he insinuated, Kinyoun spread them intentionally.

"Could it have been possible," said Gage, "that some dead body of a Chinaman had innocently *or otherwise* received a post-mortem inoculation in a lymphatic region by some one possessing the imported plague bacilli, and that honest people were thereby deluded?"[20]

Before, Kinyoun was a bumbling sorcerer's apprentice. Now, he was a mad scientist spiking corpses with bubonic germs.

To defend the state from such demonic experiments, Gage proposed making it a felony to import plague bacteria, to make slides or cultures from it, or to inoculate animals with it. He also proposed making it a felony for newspapers to publish "any false report on the presence of bubonic plague."[21]

Rallying around the governor, the legislature passed a joint resolution on January 23 asking President McKinley to remove Kinyoun from West Coast duty. Fearing exile was too mild a punishment, the bill's author added that Kinyoun should be hanged.[22]

"I did not know that a man occupying such a high position as the Governor of a State, could stoop so low as to lend himself to one of the lowest forms of persecution," Kinyoun wrote to his aunt and uncle. "His statements were more in keeping with what is found in the yellow-backed dime novels, than what has really occurred. . . ."[23]

After eighteen months of toil and family sacrifice on Angel Island, Kinyoun was denounced as a fraud. He wired the surgeon general, asking to be avenged for the slander.[24]

But Kinyoun got a vote of no confidence from his boss. With federal-state relations in San Francisco frayed past repair, Wyman sent in a new man to manage the crisis. Joseph H. White was a veteran who had fought cholera in Hamburg and leprosy in Hawaii. The day after New Year's, White set down his suitcase at the Occidental Hotel on Sutter Street and set to work.

Newspapers promoted the theory that White had come to reverse Kinyoun's diagnosis. But soon after his arrival, Chung Wey Lung, a sixty-year-old merchant, died in his basement store at 720 Jackson Street.

Kinyoun took Joe White to view the unfortunate man, whom he referred to as a "low, dirty Chinese."[25] Desperate for White to believe him, he saw the dead man not as a patient, but as proof of his hypothesis.

The slides and cultures confirmed that Chung was the city's twenty-third plague victim in ten months. In marking the number 23 on the Chinatown map in pink ink—the color code for the year 1901—the public health officers saw that all but two of Chinatown's dozen square blocks were now touched by the outbreak.

Chung's case was quickly followed by more deaths, both Chinese and white. Furious at the governor's intransigence, the city health board president, J. M. Williamson, took his case to the mayor. "The Board of Health during the whole of this bitter controversy has promulgated nothing but the exact facts," he said. "A lie is a lie whether it [be] uttered by the lips of medical sycophants hovering around the gubernatorial coattails, or whether it be traced by the point of an executive pen."[26]

Confronting a hopeless impasse, Joseph White took a decisive step. He asked Surgeon General Wyman to send a panel of independent experts to determine once and for all whether plague existed in San Francisco. Meanwhile, White kept a discreet distance from the embattled Kinyoun.

Wyman agreed, and chose his experts with care: From the University of Pennsylvania, he tapped Simon Flexner, a bespectacled thirty-seven-year-old medical educator who would later gain fame at the Rockefeller Institute in New York. From the University of Michigan, he chose Frederick Novy, thirty-six, a goateed professor of medicine. From the University of Chicago, he recruited Lewellys Barker, thirty-three, a lanky young anatomy professor who had been a protégé of the legendary William Osler at Johns Hopkins University. All three knew plague when they saw it. Novy had studied plague in Berlin. Flexner had researched it in the Philippines with Barker. Barker had then followed pestilence to Bombay, India, a city he found "preternaturally quiet and dismal" under the smoky pall of funeral pyres. There, he later wrote, he "realized what the horrors of the Black Death of Europe in earlier centuries must have been."[27]

In late January 1901, the three plague experts left their laboratories and classrooms behind and boarded trains for the West Coast. They traveled fast and light, carrying no lab equipment with them, checked into the Occidental Hotel, and looked for a laboratory where they could work. It seemed simple enough, but nothing in San Francisco was simple.

Kinyoun's laboratory on Angel Island was well equipped but tainted by controversy. A University of California scientist offered lab space but was forced to withdraw his offer for fear Governor Gage would cut his university's funding.[28]

Finally, the city of San Francisco found makeshift lab space in room 161 of City Hall. Every day, the special commission made the rounds of Chinatown, visiting the sick and the dead. Accompanying them was Wong Chung, the secretary of the Chinese Six Companies, acting as their translator and guide.

Wong Chung was a moon-faced gentleman who wore the traditional queue. A respected figure on the Chinatown commercial scene, Wong was also fluent in English, and could unlock his neighborhood's secrets as only a native speaker of Chinese could. It is hard to know what persuaded him to help the visiting doctors. Perhaps the Chinese Six Companies wanted him to inform them of what the Caucasian physicians were up to. Perhaps Wong himself suspected that the plague scare might turn out to be real. Whatever the interior thoughts of this quiet man, his work assisting the two-week investigation set the stage for a relationship between Chinese and whites that would turn the tide of the epidemic.

Every day, they improvised autopsies in dimly lit apartments, surrounded by the grieving families and friends of the dead. Then they returned to room 161 of City Hall, armed with their autopsy samples. After placing the samples on glass slides and peering into the microscope, they wrote up each case for their report.

Plague or no plague, whatever the panel found was destined for a confidential report to the surgeon general in Washington, D.C. During two weeks in February 1901, they examined thirteen people dying of all causes.

"Of the thirteen deaths which came to our attention, occurring from Feb. 5 to Feb. 16th inclusive, six were undoubtedly due to infection with plague," the panel concluded. "A seventh may have been a case of plague which went unrecognized."[29]

Among them were two actors, a theater cook, and a cigar maker who tried to soothe his buboes with a plaster of salve and honey. There was a little girl initially misdiagnosed with typhoid, and a middle-aged laborer. All had succumbed under the eyes of the nation's preeminent infectious disease specialists. Such was the power of plague and the powerlessness of doctors to stop it.

The mystery of the seventh case involved Chung Moon Woo Shee, a homemaker who died of a suspicious fever. But just as the trio of experts made the first incision in their autopsy, her watching family cried out inconsolably. Their wails of grief froze the doctors' scalpel in their hands. Out of respect, they laid down their tools. There would be no autopsy that day. Her case remained unsolved.

Just as the commission wrapped up its report, the youngest commissioner, Lewellys Barker, developed a sudden fever. He was overtaken by aches, and odd lumps began to erupt. After two weeks in plague houses and makeshift morgues, it looked ominous. They'd all taken precautions, injecting themselves with liberal doses of Yersin's plague antiserum, but it wasn't perfect protection.

Even though Yersin's antiserum was far safer than the Haffkine vaccine, it also could cause problems. The two products worked differently in the body. The preventive Haffkine vaccine, made from killed plague bacteria, was injected before exposure to immunize a person—that is, to spark the production of human antibodies that could fight off plague. The Yersin antiserum, on the other hand, was a solution of ready-made antibodies given to boost immunity even after a person was already exposed to plague. But since this antiserum was drawn from the blood of horses exposed to the plague, it contained proteins foreign to the human body. So some recipients of the antiserum mounted an intense immune reaction against these horse proteins. The reaction—fever, joint pain, and hives—was known as "serum sickness."

Serum sickness could be very dangerous indeed, but it wasn't plague. And to his colleagues' intense relief, Barker's illness turned out to be just that—a case of serum sickness mimicking early symptoms of plague. It was a false alarm, but a reminder that no one was immune.[30]

Their grim task completed, and their lips sealed about their findings, the expert panel trio prepared to leave for home. But a trickle of leaks about the plague report in the *Sacramento Bee* alerted Governor Gage to impending trouble. He demanded an audience at the Palace Hotel.

Billing his visit as a courtesy call, Gage brought a delegation and prepared to lobby the scientists to head off any threat to his state. The plague commissioners, in no mood to be bullied, gave it to him straight: The state had the plague, and they intended to report it to the surgeon general. The governor retreated to Sacramento to plot his next move.[31]

On February 28, he summoned newspaper and railroad executives. They chartered a special train to the capital and huddled with the governor until four A.M. Then, their plan of action decided, they went home to pack for Washington, D.C.[32]

Sidelined, Kinyoun watched helplessly. He tried to forewarn Surgeon General Wyman about the governor's delegation and its rumored mission to suppress the panel's findings.[33] Now in charge, Joseph White dined with the mayor and medics to muster support for his plague-control operations. But privately, he despaired. "The people and the place here," he wrote the surgeon general, "are a law unto themselves. . . ."[34]

"The situation here is worse than you think," he added. "I cannot foretell the outcome, but I fear disaster. A year ago it might have been checked but now I am extremely doubtful of any success. . . . I fear the service has met . . . a Waterloo."[35]

Seal of Silence

ON A TRAIN BOUND FOR Washington, D.C., the governor's men vowed to defend the Golden State in a deal that was pure brass. Having failed to deny the plague at home, they hoped to strike a bargain with federal officials to cover up the proof of its existence. The delegates—men from the *Chronicle,* the *Examiner,* the Union Iron Works, and the Southern Pacific Railroad—agreed with Governor Henry Gage that only secrecy could save California from the ruin of a nationwide trade embargo.

Senators George C. Perkins and Thomas R. Bard of California acted as midwives to the plan. They had wired all the parties—from Governor Gage and the newspapers to the surgeon general's bosses at the Treasury Department—to make sure everyone was on board.[1,2]

When the delegates arrived in Washington, they headed straight for a conference with Surgeon General Wyman and his bosses at the Treasury Department. California would clean up San Francisco, they promised, in exchange for a news blackout. There was no need to publicize the matter. Discretion was the key to gaining Governor Gage's cooperation with federal public health programs.

At the White House, the California delegation met with President McKinley to discuss more pleasant matters, specifically his upcoming trip to the Golden State. San Francisco had planned a lavish reception. The president and Mrs. McKinley would be guests at the Pacific Heights mansion of one of the delegates, Henry Scott, head of the

Union Iron Works. McKinley would receive tributes from the state's Republicans. He would launch one of Scott's ships. The presidential presence would advertise the state as a mecca of commerce, culture, and health. Everyone would win.

Kinyoun tried to get word to the surgeon general warning him not to trust Gage's delegates. But the sales job was a brilliant success. Surgeon General Wyman not only agreed, he asked his special plague commissioners to sign on with the plan. They acquiesced, sharing Wyman's hope that quiet diplomacy would work better than public disclosure to improve the health of San Francisco.

Wyman went further, appealing to Victor Vaughan, dean of the University of Michigan Medical School, to use his influence to discourage the Associated Press from publishing anything about the plague report. The surgeon general was worried that the wire service would break the news nationwide, and only a perfect "seal of silence" could appease California's governor, he explained.[3]

But on the anniversary of Wong Chut King's death at the old Globe, the *Sacramento Bee* broke the seal of silence. On March 6, the same day that the governor's men started for Washington, the *Bee* ran a banner headline on page one to trumpet the news of the federal panel's findings to its readers in the state capital: BUBONIC PLAGUE EXISTS IN SAN FRANCISCO. . . .[4]

But the *Bee* wasn't finished leaking plague news. In yet another page one headline, the paper next exposed the deal struck between California and the surgeon general:

**INFAMOUS COMPACT
SIGNED BY WYMAN:
MAKES AGREEMENT WITH GAGE
NOT TO LET FACTS BECOME
KNOWN CONTRARY TO
FEDERAL LAW**[5]

The story charged that the secrecy pact violated an 1893 quarantine law requiring the surgeon general to publish regular reports on the health status of U.S. ports. Concealing plague in the port of San Francisco was clearly illegal.

But Washington officials were too busy endorsing San Francisco's health to worry much. "I would feel as safe living in San Francisco as in Washington," said a top Treasury Department official. "Traveling and business can continue as safely with San Francisco today as a year ago."[6]

Kinyoun sent Wyman a telegram arguing against the compromise and predicting that the delegation from California would "promise everything and do nothing" to purge the plague.[7] When he read Kinyoun's warning wire, Wyman brusquely put the quarantine officer in his place. The deal was done, he said. Kinyoun's desire for public vindication "must be subordinated to maintain attitude of nonpublication," Wyman added. "The Department and its Officers will maintain this attitude until further orders."[8]

The lame duck quarantine officer was now muzzled as well.

But Kinyoun wasn't alone in protesting the gag order. The man who had come to replace him agreed that silence was a bad idea.

"If the facts are kept secret now," wrote Joe White to the surgeon general, "they will rise up to damn us in the future. . . ."[9]

"I am at a loss to know what you want me to do," he told the surgeon general. "This is a most peculiar situation—as I understand it, I am to say nothing about plague and yet supervise the disinfection for it," he said. But, he asked, "When I recommend moving the Chinese out of a given house and they say as they always do, 'What for?' what possible answer can be given?"[10]

Back at the University of Chicago, Lewellys Barker, who had risked his own health to verify plague in San Francisco, was uneasy with the bargain that had been struck. Besides, he wanted to see his commission's plague findings published. "The San Francisco Chronicle has been lieing [sic] shamefully lately," Barker wrote to Surgeon General Wyman on April 6.[11] There is "great dissatisfaction among many men because our full report has not been published, and the delay in publication is being misinterpreted," he said. "If the San Francisco press is still misrepresenting the situation I confess I think them no longer deserving any sympathy, after what they were told by you in Washington. It is a grave reflection upon their honesty."[12]

Even though the death toll was still relatively low, Barker wasn't complacent about San Francisco's safety. He saw too much similarity with other epidemic zones. In Hong Kong, Calcutta, and Bombay, he had seen the "sneaking progress" of a smoldering plague suddenly flare into a violent outbreak with heavy casualties.[13] He feared the worst days might lie ahead.

Back at the University of Michigan, his fellow plague commissioner Frederick Novy was thrust into an emergency after a deadly lab accident. Novy had carried vials containing bubonic plague samples from San Francisco back to Ann Arbor to grow cultures for vaccine production. He assigned star medical student Charles B. Hare to help with bacterial cultures. Having a reputation for careful technique, Hare was the only student allowed to handle bubonic plague. Hare denied having any lab accident. But somehow—perhaps because he was a smoker who rolled his own cigarettes—a droplet of the germ culture contaminated the medical student.

On the night of April 3, Hare's back began to ache and an odd sensation of numbness crept over him. Overnight, his temperature shot up to 103. Toward morning, he was convulsed by nausea. Later, he began to cough up flecks of mucus streaked with blood. Novy tested it: It was pneumonic plague.

Hare was taken to the pesthouse in a horse-drawn ambulance. His room was sealed and doused with formaldehyde. Novy wired the surgeon general for an emergency shipment of fifty bottles of Yersin's antiserum. Pneumonic plague, he knew, was the quickest killer and the toughest to treat. After injecting Hare with copious amounts of antiserum, Novy could only wait and hope.[14]

Hare's fever hit 105.5, and he sank into delirium. His roommate was isolated with him but against all odds remained well. Then, as Yersin's antiserum took effect, Hare's temperature started to subside one degree at a time. Convalescence was slow, but after a month of isolation, Hare was discharged on a stretcher. He finished medical school and went on to practice medicine in California until his death at fifty. But for the remainder of his life, he required twelve hours of bed rest a day; his heart was permanently damaged by the toxin of the plague bacteria.[15]

Plague may not have jeopardized the medical career of C. B. Hare, but it mortally wounded the career of Joseph Kinyoun. Amid strident demands for his firing, Kinyoun wired the surgeon general, asking for a couple of weeks' leave to restore his health and visit his family.

Instead of a vacation, Kinyoun received a blow. "You are hereby directed to transfer the public property under your charge to Assistant surgeon L. L. Lumsden, who has been directed to relieve you. . . . You will proceed to Detroit, Michigan, and assume charge of the Service at that station. . . ."[16]

He was given three weeks to pack up his family and get to Detroit. No thanks, no acknowledgment of service under difficult conditions— nothing was offered to soften the blow. It was just the blunt, military-style transfer favored by Dr. Wyman and the U.S. Marine Hospital Service.

Kinyoun reeled. "The orders were simply without . . . any explanation," he wrote to his relatives in the East. "I have been made the scapegoat."[17]

Wyman wanted the quarantine officer to make a quick and quiet departure, but retreat was not in Kinyoun's repertoire. Against Wyman's wishes, Kinyoun went on the offensive, making speeches at state and county medical societies about plague. He took the advantage on such occasions to take some parting shots at his enemies.

Aiming at the San Francisco doctors who wrote false death certificates, Kinyoun mocked their misdiagnosis of plague as chicken cholera. He joked that they'd actually discovered a new disease, which Kinyoun called "cholera du Chink." From his once high-minded defense of bacteriology, he had sunk to low puns and crude racial slurs.[18]

San Francisco bade a bizarre farewell to Kinyoun. On the eve of his departure from San Francisco, police came to Angel Island to arrest him for attempted murder. The charge dated from an incident five months earlier in the cold waters off Angel Island. Back in November 1900, a deaf-mute fisherman was mistaken for an escapee from military detention and fired upon by soldiers. Kinyoun claimed he had rowed out to save the man, not to assault him. But now he was accused of pulling the trigger.

"I did not fire the shots," he protested. "It is an outrage to arrest me." Since he was a federal employee, Kinyoun refused to be taken into custody by anyone but a U.S. marshal. Eventually the court dropped the charges.[19]

As he packed up his family for Detroit, Kinyoun suffered recurrent bouts of paralyzing stomach pain. Gut roiling, he asked for emergency sick leave to treat his "appendicitis." Once the pain subsided, he planned a research trip to Asia to study plague, unable to let go of his obsession with the disease that had been his downfall.

But Kinyoun's tenure as a federal public health officer was running out. He was exhausted. He couldn't help but feel that Wyman, by failing to defend his diagnosis, had devalued his contributions to bacteriology. After his research trip to Asia, he would serve out a brief time in the Marine Hospital Service. But in his heart, he had already resigned.

Bitter in professional exile, Kinyoun wrote long, rambling letters blaming the press, the politicians, and the surgeon general, who—beginning with Kinyoun's transfer to San Francisco—sought "to simply relegate [him] to oblivion."[20]

When a friend suggested that he write his life story, Kinyoun ruefully proposed a title—*Les Misérables en Quarantaine.*[21]

New Blood

◉

FOUR MONTHS IN SAN FRANCISCO were enough to break the spirit. Hamstrung by his government's gag order, Joseph White felt helpless to cure the plague in Chinatown. The place seemed an impenetrable puzzle, hiding the quick and the dead. "You cannot imagine the conditions. I cannot write them," he wrote the surgeon general. "It would take Charles Dickens to do it." White pleaded for reinforcements.

"The difficulties here are so great that never before in our history has there been a greater need for tactful and forceful officers," he wrote, "and mediocrity is I think clean out of place."

White proposed a candidate for the job, but Surgeon General Wyman had another man in mind: thirty-three-year-old Rupert Blue, who was at that moment stationed in Milwaukee, caring for sick boatmen on Lake Michigan. White had never met Blue, but he'd heard through the service grapevine that Blue was lazy and lacked the subtlety to negotiate with the Chinese.

This job takes tact, White continued. "I learn that Blue has none and is inert beside[s]," he added. "I don't know Blue and have not a reason under Heaven to dislike him, so there is nothing personal in this matter at all, but I am fully persuaded that he cannot take the lead in this matter now or in the future."[1]

Ignoring White's doubts about his candidate, Wyman shipped

Blue his orders to leave the Milwaukee station and proceed at once to San Francisco.

While Blue was en route, pressure was building from outside the state for action. Texas health chief W. F. Blunt demanded a copy of the plague commission's report. Colorado health chief G. E. Tyler declared, "Concealment of contagious diseases is an unpardonable sin in public health work."[2] Newspapers in New York City and Washington State were beginning to sound alarms about California's cover-up.

Suddenly the gag order was violated. The *Sacramento Bee* and a western medical journal, the *Occidental Medical Times,* obtained bootleg copies of the plague commission's study from anonymous sources and rushed it into print. Surgeon General Wyman swiftly moved to eclipse the bootleg version by publishing the official special plague commission findings in the U.S. Public Health reports. At last, the word was out nationwide.[3]

Joe White, relieved to be rid of secrecy, denied he was the source of the leak and added that he didn't think Kinyoun was, either. Few but the experts on the panel and the surgeon general were privy to the report. The source of the leak was never identified.

Rupert Blue arrived in San Francisco for duty just as the city launched a frenzied beautification project in anticipation of the visit of President William McKinley. On an embankment in front of the Victorian flower conservatory in Golden Gate Park, gardeners planted a tapestry of poppies and pansies spelling out "California's Welcome to Our President," flanked by an American eagle and a California grizzly bear. Miles of bunting and millions of red-white-and-blue flags decked the parade route. Market Street was strung with electric bulbs and Chinese lanterns that shed a patriotic radiance, Asian-Pacific style.

The moment he got off the train, Blue inhaled the brine-scented fog, with undercurrents of beer and sewage he remembered from his first visit as a young assistant surgeon on quarantine duty in 1895. The city now had a few more electric lights and motorcars, but its raffish spirit was intact.

Indeed, San Franciscans were intoxicated with speed in the new century. The traditional Sunday carriage caravans through Golden Gate Park were now joined by two dozen rattletrap horseless carriages, tearing through town at fifteen miles an hour. But neither time nor technology had tamed the Barbary Coast, Blue found as he stepped off the train and into a tug-of-war over a corpse.

The corpse was that of a man named Mark Quan Wing. The Chinatown resident had been suffering from tuberculosis—on that, everyone agreed. But the knot of swollen glands under his armpit looked like bubonic plague. Could the two infections coexist? Joseph White demanded a test. Governor Gage's state health board ridiculed him. "It seems to make no difference then if a Chinaman died with consumption," huffed a doctor working for the state. "He has got to have buboe and clap, gallstones, appendicitis and everything else just to satisfy some people."[4]

"It is an ugly state of affairs," Joseph White brooded. The state earmarked $25,000 of its $100,000 plague fund for cleaning Chinatown. But so far the state doctors' main job seemed to be disputing a plague diagnosis.

There was one bright spot, White reported. "Blue is coming out much stronger . . . than I had thought possible," he wrote to Washington. "He has done some very good things through self-control and apparently imperturbable good nature."[5]

In the midst of the wrangling, he remained unbruised. He didn't engage the state board and the Chinese head-on. With a genial smile beneath his signature mustache, Blue gave all sides the impression that he saw their respective points. Joseph White had to admit that the unflattering gossip about Blue had been wrong.

But just as Blue arrived to help White clean Chinatown, a mysterious pause in plague cases occurred. Joseph White had his suspicions. "The cases shown to us and the corpses brought to us for examination after death have distinctly the appearance of having been culled," he reported to the surgeon general. The sick people he was allowed to see suffered from cancer and other chronic ailments; he never saw any acute cases of fever. It was strange for a population of Chinatown's size. "These people," he said, "do not wish us to find plague."[6]

Poring over death records for Chinatown, White was struck by the plunge in mortality figures to a fraction of the normal toll. "I feel sure that they are hiding the dead," he told Wyman. So with the chief of police, he plotted a new strategy. The police would conduct raids on gambling dens. Once inside, they would look around for sick people, and they would let White know the results. It was a desperate ploy to reach beyond the few cases he saw that the state doctors had handpicked for him.[7]

Were bodies stowed beneath the sidewalk? Were they spirited out of the city under cover of darkness? White sent a telegram to Washington requesting authority to fan out around San Francisco for a radius of one hundred miles, in the hope of tracking down missing cases.[8]

While White wrangled, Blue dug in to inspect the blocks around Dupont Street for sanitary problems. He found cellars afloat with sewage and vermin, the result of years of landlord neglect.

Poking about a garbage heap in back of the store owned by Sing Fah on Dupont Street, Blue was appalled. Sing Fah's was the finest store in Chinatown, stocking elegant Asian imports. But behind it, Blue found squalor. He recoiled upon discovering a garbage dump with about 150 pounds of rotten meat hidden underneath it.[9]

Still, they found no plague cases among the trickle of Chinese patients they were allowed to see. State-appointed doctors, meanwhile, insisted on being consulted each time the federal officers disinfected a house or fumigated a sewer. Finally, White could take no more. He fired off a furious letter to the governor, charging his medical team with concealment.

The tally of sick and dead was "ridiculously . . . preposterously out of proportion" with a community of Chinatown's size, he wrote.[10] He surmised that the sick and dead were being whisked across the bay to Oakland or as far away as Sacramento, one hundred miles to the east. Meanwhile, when White did manage to see a body, Gage's men would appear at the morgue, demanding tissue samples, arguing over the meaning of symptoms, and pressing competing diagnoses that were naïve or downright fraudulent.

White was fed up. He wrote Wyman that the governor, after promising Washington to clean up Chinatown, had "complied with the meagre letter of the agreement, but not in its full spirit" of plague eradication.[11]

Moreover, White heard that as soon as six weeks had passed without a new case, Governor Gage planned to declare the plague over and end the campaign. That date—June 9—was fast approaching. White urged Surgeon General Wyman not to make a dishonorable peace with the state. The service should refuse to issue a false certificate of health to the city. It would be better to pull its men out of the state and simply "allow California to work out her own destiny."[12]

Throughout this war of nerves, Blue didn't seem to get riled—by the obstructionism of the state or the passive resistance of the Chinese. He deflected attacks rather than battering opponents head-on. Beneath his charming facade, he was a soldier's son and a tactician.

White now saw the young officer as a potential successor, one who could free him to return to the East Coast. "Regarding Blue," White reported to Washington. "His work to date has been most excellent. . . . The impression [that] he was not a man of pronounced personality and executive ability, although a very nice gentleman, is utterly erroneous. He has untangled a good many rather difficult snarls; has an immense amount of self-possession and good temper, and is altogether fully capable of acting as executive officer. . . ."[13]

White's endorsement helped Blue win a promotion. In later years, White might have felt regret. Blue would one day be his rival for high office.

San Franciscans—most oblivious to the plague intrigues—were fixated on a different medical drama. President McKinley arrived on May 13 in a San Francisco decked with bouquets and bunting. But the figure that emerged from the presidential Pullman coach looked not like the commander in chief people expected, but rather like the worried consort of a gravely ill First Lady.[14] A string of daily bulletins, hinting at typhoid, said her death was near.

Banquets were canceled and bouquets wilted as Mrs. McKinley remained in a sickbed at the Scott mansion on Laguna and Clay Streets. The president scrapped most of his schedule. Citizens who lined the streets to cheer instead raised their hats and handkerchiefs in a silent salute. After receiving doses of heart stimulants, Mrs. McKinley rallied and returned with her husband to the East Coast.[15]

Granted his wish to return to Washington, Joseph White also left San Francisco in early June. Staying on to oversee the floundering plague campaign was Rupert Blue—assisted by two other officers.

California's governor, as predicted, declared plague nonexistent and pulled his money out of San Francisco in June, leaving the federal doctors and the city holding the reins. Blue optimistically forecast that he would complete the hygienic and sanitary overhaul of

Chinatown on June 22. But he also quietly set up headquarters that would serve as the nerve center for a much longer siege. He leased a morgue and laboratory for $75 a month on Merchant Street, a small alley near Chinatown's Portsmouth Square. He was in business.

There was still the delicate matter of the disappearing corpses. Blue proposed that the federal government run its own hearse service. He asked the surgeon general for $35 a month to rent a horse, cart, and driver as the only way to prevent "surreptitious removals or substitution of bodies."[16] Dr. Wyman agreed but promised Governor Gage that Dr. Blue and two assistants would be around just a little while longer.[17] He had only a skeleton staff to conduct what Wyman implied was a phaseout of the unpopular plague operation. Dr. Mark J. White inspected the sick, and Dr. Donald H. Currie ran the morgue and lab.

With public health threats apparently under control, San Franciscans now reclined into summer like it was a hammock. The upper class left for resorts in San Rafael or Santa Cruz. In town, *Aïda* opened the summer season at the Tivoli Opera House.

Just after Independence Day 1901, plague returned in a corner of Chinatown's demimonde. Blue and his men had just finished testing the corpse of an asparagus harvester for plague on the night of Monday, July 8, and were washing off the smell of the lab, possibly looking forward to a drink, when the calls came. There was a cluster of fever breaking out in a Chinatown crib.

A Japanese physician, Dr. Kurozawa, was the first to arrive at the apartment at 845 Washington Street. The Yoshiwara House was a Japanese brothel in the heart of the Chinese quarter. It had a stable of seven women catering to an Asian and a citywide clientele. That night, three of its women—Miyo, Shina, and Ume—lay prostrate with fever and pain.

Under their kimonos, Shina and Miyo had egg-size lumps protruding from their pelvises. The third patient, Ume, had a tender swelling under her right arm. Alarmed, Dr. Kurozawa called a network of city physicians, who called the bacteriologist H. A. L. Ryfkogel. Ryfkogel alerted Rupert Blue.

All natives of Japan in their mid-twenties, the women had worked at Yoshiwara House for about one year. In late Victorian parlance, such women were called "inmates"—their profession was a life sentence. Some were sold by impoverished families, others accepted passage to America for a job that turned out to be in the flesh trade. Most died young, drained and disfigured by disease.

Ryfkogel and the city health board rushed to the scene, followed by Blue and his men. The city doctors slapped a quarantine on the house, holding the other inmates for observation until Ryfkogel could make a diagnosis. Terrified of quarantine, a girl called Fuku Inaki slipped downstairs and ran four blocks away to a house on Pine Street.

The men proceeded to examine the three prostitutes. The symptoms looked like classic plague, but clinical impressions weren't enough to confirm a diagnosis. Ryfkogel drew blood samples from Shina, Miyo, and Ume and hopped a streetcar back to his lab on Sutter Street. Confirmatory cultures and animal inoculation tests would take days. Until then, he could do a kind of quick antibody test called an agglutination reaction. In it, he mixed the girls' blood with plague bacteria cultured in bouillon. If particles in the fluid clumped together, plague was present. The mix curdled into clots. "Immediate and characteristic," Ryfkogel noted. The test "makes it absolutely certain that the three suffered from the same disease and this disease was bubonic plague."[18]

Finding the culprit didn't change the women's fate; their illness was far too advanced for treatment. Just hours after they were examined, Shina and Miyo slipped into a coma. With their lymph glands hemorrhaging, the plague toxin raced through their bloodstream. Their blood pressure plunged, and shock set in. The ebony pools of their pupils were frozen, fixed and dilated. Around three A.M. on July 9, the two women died. Their colleague Ume, seething with a fever of 105, wasn't expected to live.

At twelve noon, Miyo's shrouded form was carried to the morgue on Commercial Street for autopsy. In attendance were federal and city physicians, with the state doctors hovering to quibble over points of lab technique. The federal doctors donned rubber aprons and began their barehanded autopsy of Miyo, a twenty-six-year-old female, stiffened by rigor mortis. The doctors made a long median incision from sternum to pubis, opened her peritoneum, pushed aside coils of viscera, and found the knot of inflamed lymph glands in her right pelvis. Her spleen was swollen to twice the normal size. The doctors carefully extracted bits of tissue to grow in culture.[19]

At three P.M., they began the autopsy of Shina, also just twenty-six. She was "a well-developed and well-nourished young woman," with an unblemished complexion and no sign of venereal disease. After carving carefully around the buboes in her left and right pelvis, the doctors eased out the skein of inflamed lymph glands, which oozed blood.[20]

With the naked eye, they would later watch as cultures made from those samples, smeared across agar plates, developed into germ colonies with the classic "ground glass" texture of plague. Under the microscope, the colonies were made up of the short-rounded rods of plague bacteria. And the guinea pigs injected with the cultures developed the same swollen glands, the same fatal outcome.

Now Blue began using the health service codebook to wire the test results to Surgeon General Wyman: "Bumpkin malleate . . ."[21] Plague diagnosis confirmed.

About the time her co-workers lay cooling on the autopsy slab, young Ume surprised the doctors by rebounding. Blue declared her to be the first patient ever to survive plague in San Francisco.

But the case of the fugitive Fuku Inaki was hopeless. Health officers caught up with the young prostitute on Pine Street and brought her back to the brothel in Chinatown for observation. The Chinese press protested her return to Chinatown as proof the federal doctors wished them ill and sought to concentrate all the plague in their neighborhood.[22] By July 11, she was dead. Kimonos and bedding used by the Yoshiwara women were piled in the street and burned.

Blue's next task was to worry about the men who had patronized the brothel. It wouldn't be easy. Before they fell ill, Blue estimated, the women had serviced at least fifty men between them, and so far not a single case of suspicious illness had been reported. "Truly an anomaly," he puzzled.[23]

Blue watched his men rushing from brothel to morgue, and morgue to laboratory, hastily disinfecting their equipment in between cases as best they could. With the fumes of formaldehyde and carbolic acid still singeing his nostrils, Blue hinted that the task was more than Wyman had envisioned. To protect themselves, the men were injecting each other regularly with Yersin's plague antiserum. It was expensive, and it carried the same risks of serum sickness that had troubled Lewellys Barker. But as they were constantly being exposed to plague germs without the modern protection of latex gloves and face shields, it was their only option.

The outbreak also tested Blue's diplomacy. "Much hard feeling has been engendered over these cases between Bursary [the code word for the California State Health Board] on the one side and Burlesque [the San Francisco Health Board] and Ryfkogel on the other," he wrote. "Our laboratory technique has been unfairly criticised by [the state physician] Dr. Mathews, and I found it very hard to refrain a retort in kind. There is so much at stake, and as we are only seeking the truth, I shall always try to maintain a friendly relationship with them. . . . We have borne a good deal and can bear a great deal more for the good of the Service and the cause."[24]

Blue had run into the same wall of denial and deceit that had bedeviled Joseph Kinyoun and Joseph White. Now those forces were obstructing his mission, complaining about the lab assistance of Drs. Kellogg and Ryfkogel. However, Blue's way was not to collide head-on, but rather to circumvent.

"I humored them to the extent of saying that only our Service men should touch or handle preparations in the laboratory. I did this with a view to forestall any unjust criticism that might be given out by them. Of course, I know that Doctors Ryfkogel and Kellogg are as safe to have around as any men in the profession, but I did not want our work discredited on account of local prejudice," he reported to Washington. "There is some amusement to be gained by yielding to some of their objections, for then we are put on the *qui vive*."[25] A soldier's son, Blue remained on the alert, on the qui vive, a French sentry's cry that means "Who goes there?"

Despite five new cases and four deaths, the newspapers largely ignored the outbreak, and most San Franciscans were oblivious to any hazard that might spoil their summer. Even Ho Yow, the consul of China, took a break from his diplomatic duties in August to attend the summer harness races in the hotbox of Sacramento. There, his mare Solo streaked ahead of the competition. Sore losers attributed Solo's victory to her driver's racing silks, with their coiled dragon, which mesmerized the competition.

The city's long-festering labor unrest exploded in late summer. By a unanimous vote of the City Labor Federation, a general strike was called on July 29. City teamsters were idled, along with fifteen thousand sailors, longshoremen, and freight handlers on the waterfront. The port was paralyzed. Striking workers marched four abreast down Market Street. By August, the strike funds and patience were running out.

On August 28, as five hundred striking teamsters left a benefit baseball game south of Market Street, they ran into dray wagons driven by nonunion men. Hurling rocks, the strikers harried the strikebreakers up 6th Street to Market. The rioters were cheered by five thousand spectators. Special police fired guns to break up the mob. Scores were bloodied in the melee, but no one was killed.[26]

Plague, however, was still a lethal force. Its next assault occurred in late August, just as Chinatown celebrated a festival of the dead. People donned their fine silk robes. The streets were hung with lanterns and bouquets. Scrolls of poetry were burned, and tables of delicacies were spread out to propitiate the souls of the departed. The very next day they had a new spirit to appease.

On August 31, the body of a twenty-eight-year-old Chinese man, Lee Mon Chou, was carried to the plague morgue. Lee had an infection that ruptured glands in his pelvis and invaded his lungs. He died at the Oso Cigar Factory on Dupont Street, where he worked among a dozen men. With a cough or a sneeze, Lee could have infected them all. The cigar factory was immediately shut down, fumigated with sulfur, and swabbed with formaldehyde. But before the doctors could find the dead man's co-workers, they disappeared like wisps of incense from a joss stick.[27]

Just before Labor Day, Blue boarded a train out of San Francisco to settle some personal business, leaving the Merchant Street morgue and lab in the able hands of Mark White and Donald Currie. The bullying of the plague doctors intensified in his absence. For the first time, San Franciscans opened their papers to read about some unorthodox uses of Governor Gage's plague fund.

The Morse Detective Agency billed the state health board $326.25 for spying on the bacteriologist H. A. L. Ryfkogel and the federal doctors as they made their rounds in Chinatown. They insinuated that Ryfkogel was inoculating Chinese corpses with plague, as they had said Kinyoun was. "Governor Gage has not the instincts of a gentleman," Ryfkogel told the local press. "I am not a bit surprised to hear that he had my footsteps dogged through Chinatown by hired shadows."[28]

But any outrage brewing over the state-funded spying was immediately eclipsed by the report of gunshots three thousand miles away. In Buffalo, New York, while President William McKinley attended a reception inside the Temple of Music at the Pan-American Exposition, an anarchist named Leon Czolgosz rushed up and pumped two bullets into his chest and abdomen. McKinley remained conscious, prayed aloud, comforted his wife, and bade the American people to keep courage. For eight days he fought, but he ultimately succumbed to his wounds.

At 2:15 A.M. on September 14, San Francisco fire stations tolled, ringing fifty-eight times, once for every year of McKinley's life. Stricken crowds gathered outside the newspaper offices and numbly absorbed the news. Behind his wire rims, the newspapers said, the newly sworn forty-two-year-old President Theodore Roosevelt fought back tears.

Rupert Blue headed back to San Francisco just in time to tie on a black crepe armband for the month of mourning ordered by Surgeon General Wyman.

The Bite of a Flea

◉

COOPED UP IN RAILROAD CARS for two weeks, Blue was restless and itching to get back to the plague lab and morgue on Merchant Street. After his brief personal leave, he seemed eager to plunge back into the fray and forget his own troubles. "Work of any kind, after such an experience, would [be] a blessing," he told the surgeon general.[1]

His life with Juliette was unraveling. Since their marriage in 1895, they had moved nine times for the federal health service. The life of a circuit-riding sanitarian—as rootless as a soldier's, but without the status—was rough on families. Now, seven years later, the nomadic life, with its constant transfers, modest pay, and no permanent home, took its toll. If Rupert and Juliette's marriage in 1895 didn't give his mother the vapors, then their breakup certainly did. Divorce was scandalous in his church and his state. But despite the stigma, their union ended in 1902. After they parted, all traces of Julie—as he once affectionately called her—disappeared from his life. No letters, pictures, or mementos of the young actress he loved survive in his family's records or correspondence, as if purging her name would efface the shame of divorce.

Blue would immerse himself in the plague zone. He had a lot of catching up to do; the men had been very busy in his absence. But at least the team now had a Chinese translator.

Before he had left San Francisco, Joe White had tried to hire

Wong Chung, the Chinese Six Companies' old secretary, to act as the Marine Hospital Service interpreter for the then substantial wage of $5 a day. Wong had been a key to the success of the independent plague commission. Guiding the men through Chinatown, he opened up access that only a native speaker could provide. But apparently the interpreter wasn't eager to work with the white doctors as a steady job—not yet, anyway. After White's overture, Wong Chung shied away, left town, and stayed incommunicado for several weeks.

But federal doctors intensified their courtship and overcame Wong Chung's reluctance. Wong took the job. After his brief stint as translator for the visiting plague experts in early 1901, he now expanded his role into that of regular translator for the Washington doctors. Translators in that day wore many hats, from simple interpreter to cultural emissary to negotiator with the whites. (Indeed, one term for translator, *cheut faan*, literally means one who goes "out to the barbarians.")[2] So it's likely that Wong's access to federal health officials helped keep Chinatown leaders informed of Washington's next move against the plague. However, it's also likely that Wong now saw that plague wasn't merely the invention of white racists, or a pretext for a crackdown on Chinatown, but a dangerous disease that imperiled his people. Whatever his private motives for taking the job, it was a role that carried heavy personal risks—the risk of being censured by the state, and shunned by his own kind.

The translator was proving to be a font of medical and political intelligence. Wong tipped off the federal doctors that a clerk was sick in the basement of Fook Lung & Company, a Washington Street grocery. Mark White—not to be confused with Joseph White—set out to investigate. Languishing in a basement bunk beneath the sidewalk, twenty-eight-year-old Ng Chan burned and shivered with a fever of over 103 degrees. The walnut-size lump in his groin conformed with the clinical picture of plague. It seemed clear-cut.

But not to the doctors of the state health board, who called it venereal disease and advised Ng Chan not to cooperate with the federal physicians. Ng denied requests for a blood test or a photograph of his bubo. At the Oriental Dispensary, he received visitors, five and six at a time, who chatted at his bedside as if he had a cold.

One evening during visiting hours, the friends of Ng Chan hatched a plot to smuggle the patient to a Sacramento River ranch—

with help from the state health board. A hospital janitor let in on the scheme slipped word to Wong Chung. Wong alerted Mark White, who posted guards at the bedside, foiling the getaway.

Spiriting sick people away to the country had to be prevented, or all plague measures would be for naught. But Mark White was aware that the situation was delicate. If he were punitive or disparaging, as Kinyoun had been, he'd lose the trust and goodwill of the people. "I do not think the Chinese here very different from the Human Race elsewhere," he wrote to Washington. By treating people with respect, he added, public health goals "can be far more readily attained."[3] It was a simple observation, but radical for its day.

The city's rats continued to gnaw through the illusory wall separating whites and Asians. Their next victim was a middle-aged white seaman. Alexander Winters, a fifty-year-old salt, toiled aboard small schooners and scows from San Francisco Bay to the Sacramento River Delta. He'd never had anything more than a case of clap in his youth.

"I made one trip on the *Agnes Jones* up to Rio vista to get hay, which was unloaded at the foot of Third Street, San Francisco," he told Rupert Blue. "About September 9th, while still in the vessels, I had a very heavy chill, with headache, fever and vomiting, and at the same time I noticed the bubo in my groin. It was very painful and interfered with walking. . . .

"On the next day, I went ashore, when I was sick two days and thought I would surely kick the bucket," Winters told Blue.[4]

Winters lived to tell his story. But his case only confounded the doctors. By the time he got sick, his ship had sailed away. The federal team traced his steps back to the France House, a sailors' hostel at 149 3rd Street. They found the other boarders healthy.

Blue was stumped. Winters had had no contact with Chinatown, so his case hinted at a far wider plague infestation than previously thought. "I would rather find a Chinese origin for this case, than to think that the sailors' haunts on the waterfront were infected," Blue told Surgeon General Wyman. Since the waterfront harbored as many rats as Chinatown, plague there would be disastrous. "If we have then the two worst sections of the city infected," he said, "eradication of the disease is entirely out of the question, and the danger of an indefinite stay is enhanced."[5]

Before Blue could solve the mystery of Alex Winters's plague, the sickness struck again.

Marguerete Saggau was a fifty-three-year-old matron who lived at the Hotel Europa on Broadway. Mrs. Saggau was a laundress. Her husband and son were teamsters who hauled goods in and out of Chinatown. But on September 23, Mrs. Saggau swooned, vomited, and developed shaking chills. The next day, her head throbbed, her temperature soared, and her senses wandered.

On admission at German Hospital, she had a fever of 103 degrees. After palpating the lump in her pelvis, they put Mrs. Saggau in isolation. But by September 27, she was dead, and the desperate detective work began anew. "It would not be an easy matter to trace the source of this infection," Blue told Washington for the second time that week. Her teamster husband and son were healthy. Her laundry customers at the Hotel Europa were, too. So he ruled out Chinese goods and soiled linen as sources of infection.

"Then," Blue wrote his boss, "the Hotel Europa, where the family lived, is only one block north of Chinatown, a distance easily covered by rats in their migration. . . ."[6]

Here at last was a clue that meant something. Perhaps Mrs. Saggau's fatal infection didn't come from Chinese wares or dirty laundry, or food or dust. The agents of infection couldn't be fenced or quarantined, because they were mobile, sequestered in the walls, slipping in stealth from house to house.

Sick rats had been seen as the harbingers of plague for centuries. However, their link with human casualties remained a mystery. But then Paul-Louis Simond, a Pasteur Institute scientist working in India, theorized that plague in rats and people had a common cause. Simond suspected that the missing link was *la piqûre de puce*—the bite of a flea. He conducted a simple but elegant experiment in 1897. He installed two rats in separate cages side by side. One had plague, the other was healthy. The cages prevented physical contact between the two rodents, but their open grillwork let the fleas hop back and forth. When the plague rat died, the fleas deserted its corpse and jumped through the bars to the healthy rat in the neighboring cage. As they sucked blood from their new host, they injected plague bacteria. Within six days, the second rat died, too, its blood brimming with plague.[7]

Unhappily for patients yet to come, Simond's breakthrough only drew scorn from medical skeptics. Plague was still seen as a scourge of dark-skinned aliens. These prejudices persisted until 1906, when the British plague commission in India confirmed Simond's findings. Only then would the medical establishment accept flea-borne transmission as the spark of deadly plague epidemics.

When San Francisco's plague struck in 1900, Simond's flea discovery was three years old. Scientists in Sydney that year gave the theory added credence by discovering plague bacteria in the stomach of fleas. The explosive impact of these findings, when taken together, was swamped in a sea of lesser theories.

Surgeon General Walter Wyman had published his own monograph on plague in January 1900. In it, he reviewed a host of hypotheses. Plague, he said, can be contracted by inhaling dust, consuming tainted food or drink, and handling contaminated household goods. In citing a successful German rat bounty, where people were paid 5 pfennig apiece for dead rodents, Wyman neared an insight.

"It is very possible that the fleas which infest rats, and which notoriously leave their bodies as soon as the cadavers become cold after death, may by their bites infect other rats," he wrote. But after coming so close to the heart of the matter, Wyman retreated. "The bites of insects play a very small role," he concluded.[8] In the end, the surgeon general endorsed the racial theory of plague as a disease that selectively attacked Asians, owing to their poverty and vegetarian diets.

Meanwhile, San Francisco rats bred and spread, heedless of skin color or scientific fashion.

Wong Chung, Detective

◈

RED CIRCLES AND BLACK CROSSES multiplied across the map of Chinatown, marking new cases and deaths. The city health board tried to help, but the state health board blocked Blue at every turn.

Dr. W. P. Mathews, secretary of the state health board, burst into the Merchant Street lab, loudly declaring that the federal doctors had no authority to practice medicine in California. If they kept on diagnosing plague, he threatened, he'd cut off their access to patients.

Blue exploded. "Scant courtesy, singular apathy, and in the end, interference have characterized [the state board] at a time of grave public peril," he wrote to Surgeon General Wyman.[1]

In the face of state hostility, Blue told Wyman he was relying more and more on his interpreter, Wong Chung. Wong's evolution from simple translator to disease sleuth galvanized Blue's investigation. Wong Chung helped sift fact from fiction in the most difficult cases. And the state health board wasn't happy about it.

Two physicians working in league with the state, William Lawlor and Elmer Stone, "shamefully abused" Wong Chung for reporting cases to the federal doctors, a worried Mark White told Blue. The state doctors spread word through the streets of Chinatown that federal plague doctors were only out to oppress the community. By assisting them, they added, Wong Chung had turned traitor. White said the two had warned Wong, "[S]omebody was going to get killed."[2]

There was no doubt: The Barbary Coast turned the public health canon on its head. Yet even in the depth of their frustration with the state, Rupert Blue and Mark White were learning that they could relax some of the most rigid protocols of quarantine. While showing no mercy to the germ of plague, they began to show more leniency toward its victims. Where Joseph Kinyoun and Joseph White had seen the Chinese as liars, Rupert Blue and Mark White saw instead a people driven from fear to evasion and from evasion into further danger.

"To remove the fear of a ruinous quarantine . . . will take away one-half the Chinaman's hostility," Blue wrote Washington. From now on he would quickly disinfect a plague house, isolate only the patient's immediate family, and reopen the place in a few days so life could return to normal. Still, suspicions died hard.

"It is almost impossible to catch the Chinese contacts," Blue admitted. "They seem to know a suspicious case, and depart, like the fleas, before the body cools off. Each case, though, is a law unto itself . . . and no rule can be set for all of them. We are still working quietly, avoiding friction with the state or the Chinese."[3]

In the same letter, Blue warned that plague was unpredictable: "The outcome of the situation here defies any attempt to outline it."

Every morning, Blue and White left the Occidental Hotel and walked or hopped a streetcar for the half a dozen blocks north toward Chinatown. A briny wind off the bay stirred morning scents of coffee, sourdough, and the deposits left by carriage horses.

When they passed the corner of Clay and Kearny, with Telegraph Hill rising ahead of them, Blue and White continued another half block north and turned into the narrow alley of Merchant Street. Once through the laboratory doors, they entered a cloud of disinfectant vapor mixed with the musky warmth of the animal lab. In autumn 1901, the morgue was receiving a steady drip of customers, and today was no exception.

The hearse driver nodded toward a shrouded figure on a litter. Lifting the sheet, Blue saw the husk of a middle-aged laborer lying still and sallow, with mumpslike swellings jutting under his jaw. Chew Ban Yuen, a forty-year-old migrant worker, had just returned from a season in the Alaska fish canneries when he was felled by a profound weakness and savage sore throat. His friends brought balms from a traditional healer—to no avail. He died September 29 in a fetid, sun-less tenement on Waverly Street. His autopsy confirmed plague.

Newspapers were full of the coming mayoral election, but plague was the issue that everyone dodged. The campaign was all about labor and management. After a summer of strike violence, San Franciscans—especially workers—were bruised and vulnerable to seduction by a new party promising a progressive labor stance. This opportunity beckoned to a political kingmaker named Abraham Ruef and his handpicked mayoral candidate, the suave society violinist Eugene Schmitz.[4]

Schmitz had never given a speech, but he was a Victorian Adonis with a lush black pompadour and beard. Ruef supplied the brains and cash for the campaign. And without ever uttering the word *plague,* the new Union Labor candidate vaulted into the lead.

From the lab on Merchant Street, the public health team watched the race with unease. As dusk fell on Election Day, November 5, crowds gathered at Kearny and Market Streets. Colored fireworks would signal the winner: red for the Democrats, white for the Republicans, and green for Labor. A brass band blared, punctuated by the boom of rockets. In a shower of sparkles that lit the crowd with the color of money, Schmitz was proclaimed mayor. Boisterous joy rocked the working-class districts south of Market Street.[5]

The joy was short-lived. Once installed, the Union Labor Party was less about principles than power. Now attorney to the mayor, Abe Ruef set about perfecting the art of graft. After hours at the Pup saloon, Ruef nursed a glass of absinthe and received lines of favor seekers, soliciting $1 million in legal retainers—bribes—from utility companies, gambling parlors, boxing clubs, and brothels.[6]

With so many rich veins of patronage to be mined, City Hall saw scant profit in public health. During the weeks surrounding the election, the rat fleas attacked and sickened seven new people in China-town. Before Christmas, a barber, a cobbler, a cigar maker, and a hardware salesman would land in the morgue.

A lucky few were like Huie Jin, who contracted a mild case of plague. Ignoring Mark White's biopsy results indicating plague, state doctors diagnosed venereal disease. When Huie Jim sued for release from quarantine, the state board of health backed his demand and helped win his release.[7]

Huie Jin survived his brush with plague. But the habeas corpus cases further frayed state-federal relations. The new mayor kept mum.

Cold weather was the off-season for plague. Sweeping in ahead of the rainy season, chill winds drove the rats underground, into warm basements and subterranean sewers. There the rat sickness would fester unseen until spring coaxed the animals back into human dwellings.

While disease wintered in the Asian quarter, white San Franciscans felt carefree. With the strikes settled and the election decided, autumn arts and sporting exhibitions took center stage. A covey of divas flocked to town for opera season. Sybil Sanderson came to star in *Manon,* and Ernestine Schumann-Heink unleashed her throaty contralto in *Die Walküre*.

After a crowd of 3,300 cheered her performance in *Lohengrin,* the soprano Emma Eames took a day off and went adventuring in Chinatown. Riding past pearl dealers and fishmongers, she soaked up its mix of splendor and squalor. She took tea at a Dupont Street restaurant, then dashed back to her Palace suite, urging her fellow singers to do Chinatown. Still unsure how the disease spread, the public health officers must have felt uneasy about tourists in a plague zone. But they kept silent about the diva's visit.

Rupert Blue liked grand opera well enough, but he spent more of his free nights on boxing than bel canto. Billed by promoters as "the arts fistic," boxing was the municipal sport. The public worshiped icons of the ring like Gentleman Jim Corbett. His mighty physique was displayed across the illustrated sports pages, along with a table of his muscle measurements. His contests in the ring and his turbulent love life were news events. Quacks sold electric belts that promised to turn weaklings into mountains of muscle.

While the silk-hatted and ermine-caped set settled into the plush tiers of the Grand Opera, a crowd of seven thousand boxing fans snaked into the cavernous Mechanics' Pavilion at Larkin and Grove Streets. For $2 to $20 a ticket, spectators could watch the favorite, Jim Jeffries, pound challenger Gus Ruhlin. The mellow gaslights dimmed. Eighty new arc lights snapped on, flooding the ring in an electric aura "more brilliant than the brightest day." Grinning and cracking his gum, Jeffries bounded over the ropes and dispatched

Ruhlin in five easy rounds. Exiting in a beery haze and crunching peanut shells underfoot, the crowd grumbled that the fight was fixed. Wrote the *Chronicle* sports reporter: "They were a disgusted lot. . . ."[8]

Blue, whose forefathers all topped six feet, was a natural heavyweight and a passionate amateur boxer. When Gentleman Jim Corbett visited San Francisco, Blue arranged to meet him.

"I can't talk you out of it," Corbett told the southerner with the black handlebar mustache. "So come on out and I'll box you." In the smell of canvas and the company of men, Blue found a tonic.[9]

Spectator or sparring partner, Blue found the fights one way to purge the frustrations of his job. Like the Jeffries-Ruhlin fight, his job was an uneven match. With only medical science on his side, Blue saw the town's politics, money, and racial polarities aligned against his cause. The odds were disheartening.

ON THANKSGIVING DAY 1901, the holiday's peace was shattered in Chinatown. A tong member stole a servant girl's bracelet and pawned it. The petty theft provoked a bloodbath between rival gangs. To be sure, Chinatown was not the only crime zone in the city, but the tong murders were held up by the white press as reason enough to renew the Chinese Exclusion Act.

Tong war casualties totaled fourteen in 1901, but plague deaths exceeded twenty that year alone. More lethal than gang violence, plague was a methodical serial killer, quietly going about its business, while polite society never spoke its name.

Warily, Chinatown watched the exclusion law campaign gain steam. The Chinese Six Companies called on every Chinese in town to donate $1 to help defeat the anti-Chinese laws. Over at the offices of the *Chung Sai Yat Po,* the Chinatown daily newspaper, editors viewed the campaign with mounting alarm. Editor Ng Poon Chew, who had covered the plague discrimination cases, now saw the nationwide threat that was looming and embarked on an East Coast crusade to try to change American minds.

Barnstorming on behalf of Chinese civil rights, Reverend Chew opened with a selection of hymns, then launched into his speech. The

United States needs Asian trade to prosper, he ventured, so it must abolish the Chinese Exclusion Act.[10] With his cropped Western haircut, clipped mustache, and starched white collar, the thirty-five-year-old Chew gave audiences a look at Chinatown they had never seen. He was neither a tong hit man, an opium addict, nor a comic-strip coolie, but an educated Chinese American professional man.

Nonetheless, few heard his message. His speeches were drowned out by insistent union demands to oust coolie labor. And that was the message that reached the White House. Unlike the crude rants of the daily press, Roosevelt's exclusion-law speech was elegant. Bound in fine brown morocco with gold lettering, the president's address said American labor must be protected from "the presence in this country of any laborers [who] represent a standard of living so depressed that they can undersell our men in the labor market and drag them to a lower level." Roosevelt concluded: "I regard it as necessary, with this end in view, to re-enact immediately the law excluding Chinese laborers, and to strengthen it."[11]

So saying, the president who dined with Booker T. Washington and lowered the black-white barrier used his bully pulpit to preach Chinese exclusion. Reverend Chew returned home defeated to a Chinatown doubly infected by epidemic and exclusion fever.

IT HAD BEEN NINE MONTHS since Rupert Blue had left his quiet post in Milwaukee, having been ordered to San Francisco to wipe out plague. Now, after performing scores of autopsies, confirming dozens of diagnoses, and conducting a cleanup of Chinatown, he had, at best, fought plague to a political stalemate. In his cool soldierly diction, he had filed weekly case reports to the surgeon general, noting the numbers of plague cases and deaths, autopsies and lab tests. Although the state blocked him at every turn, he fought to maintain a stoic sense of calm and command amid the chaos.

But as 1901 drew to a close, Blue wrote to the surgeon general acknowledging his hopes of returning to the Midwest. There, he was truly in charge. There, he could command his station on the Lake Michigan waterfront without obstruction from state politicians. By year's end, Wyman granted his wish to resume command of the Milwaukee station. However, it would prove to be only a temporary leave from the woes of San Francisco, where the plague took no holiday.

Just before New Year's Day 1902, a dead rat turned up in a Stockton Street garbage can. Like an ancient augur, Mark White split the animal in two, peered into its liver, and saw plague in the year ahead. As the New Year got under way, White was left in charge of a plague that played hide-and-seek, with stuttering outbreaks and eerie pauses.

Elsewhere, 1902 had promised to be an age of progress. Marconi forecast a world where wireless transmitters would beam messages over continents. Doctors envisioned curing cancer with invisible "X-rays." In the *Examiner* on New Year's Day 1902, San Franciscans read scientific prophecies by the novelist Jules Verne. News would be transmitted by airwaves, Verne predicted. Electricity would banish night and illuminate a twenty-four-hour workday. Only airplanes made him skeptical: Man, he said, would never fly.[12]

San Francisco's profile rose to heady heights. On Nob Hill, architects drew up plans for a stone palazzo to be called the Fairmont Hotel. Developers also unveiled a blueprint for a new steel-ribbed skyscraper on California Street: the Merchants' Exchange. All the new towers boasted that they were earthquake- and fireproof—a claim that just begged to be tested.

Chinatown lit the fuse of the Lunar New Year, but its firecrackers failed to dispel its demons. Consul Ho Yow lost his job amid charges that he spent too much time at the races and too little time fighting the exclusion laws. Katie Wong Him, a twelve-year-old schoolgirl, sought admission to the city's white schools; she was rejected owing to her race. Still, the rats ran unchecked through the neighborhood. Mark White predicted "the growing likelihood of an epidemic. . . ."[13]

Swathed in fumes of formaldehyde and carbolic acid, White ruminated in his Merchant Street laboratory over how to interpret the stop-and-start rhythm of the plague cases. Was plague eradicated and then reintroduced? Was it hiding or provoking sporadic cases that went undetected? Or was it killing people whose bodies were shipped out of town in dry goods boxes and buried on Sacramento River ranches? Most likely, he feared, all three things were happening at once.

White planned to brief the new mayor, Eugene Schmitz, and enlist City Hall in the plague fight. But he never got his chance. At five P.M. on March 25, as the sun set behind the City Hall dome, Mayor Schmitz and Abe Ruef burst into the health department, startling a doctor who was giving a vaccination.

"I have removed the present Board of Health and appointed these gentlemen as their successors," said Schmitz with a flourish toward four doctors trailing behind him. "There is no plague in the city," the mayor said. By its diagnosis, the old health board was guilty of "injury and injustice to the people and the city of San Francisco."[14] The next morning's newspapers applauded the mayor's action. A judge barred the firings because no hearings had been held. But Mayor Schmitz and Boss Ruef charged back to court to defend the purge.

Meanwhile, plague kept up a petty creeping pace.

Then, on the afternoon of May 19, the phone rang at the Chinese Six Companies. Wong Chung, the translator, answered it. A voice reported a corpse at the offices of the Horn Hong Newspaper Co. on Washington Street. The body was that of an editor, Lee Mong, aged forty-six, who had fallen dead at one P.M. The caller then turned skittish, asking for whom Wong worked.

"I work for the doctors of Washington," said Wong. At this, the caller said he needed to report the death to the state health board and the Chinese Six Companies' doctor, Elmer Stone. Then he hung up.[15]

Refusal to yield bodies, false death certificates, patients coached to keep silent—it was all part of the daily game of resistance played by the state doctors, and it had Governor Gage's fingerprints all over it.

Mark White dashed off a handwritten letter to Dr. Wyman asking for the Secret Service to help find out whether the state health board was helping to conceal Chinese bodies. "I regret [to] suspect Dr. Stone of such rascality, but I believe that he is perfectly suitable for such work."[16]

Dr. Stone's boss, Governor Gage, was just then fighting for his political life. The past year's strike violence had eroded his popularity. Now fresh scandals erupted. Gage was charged with furnishing his house with prison-made furniture. In a page one exposé in the *Call* on May 24 and 26, he was linked with a San Quentin Prison procurement fraud featuring damask linens and ladies' nightgowns—unusual goods in a jail inventory. Gage sued the *Call*. The *Call* countersued and got a bench warrant for the governor's arrest. Republicans wearied of the antics. Finally, the Southern Pacific Railroad Co.—a great engine of Republican power—abandoned Gage for a new candidate, an eye doctor from Oakland named George Pardee.[17]

Even as his political star waned, Gage was proud and unrepentant about his plague stance. His Chinatown cleanup—part of the deal he cut with the surgeon general—was done on the cheap: fumigating thirty million cubic feet of Chinatown buildings using only three hundred pounds of sulfur—a job that should have taken thirty tons. It was a sham, a show cleanup that left rats and fleas alive. Still, Gage and Dr. Stone told the federal doctors that their mission was over and "should have stopped here long ago."[18]

The federal doctors did not pull out, however. The federal public health mission was, in fact, broadening its scope. Under Walter Wyman, the name of the U.S. Marine Hospital Service was changed to the U.S. Public Health and Marine Hospital Service. Just as the plague campaign had broadened from shipboard inspection to investigation of an urban outbreak, so the service was evolving now from a corps of doctors treating sick seamen to a public health service fighting epidemics all over the country.

It was fortunate that the federal doctors stayed on the scene. For in the summer of 1902, the plague came roaring back. After months of quiet infestation, the rats emerged from hiding, coated with ravenous fleas. Suddenly, Mark White and his team had more than they could handle.

On July 12, Chin Guie, an employee of the Chinese consulate, staggered into the Oriental Dispensary. The dispensary gave comfort but delayed calling the federal doctors until Chin was in his final agony. Mark White arrived to find the man near death. In five minutes, Chin was gone. White learned that one of the state board's doctors, Dr. Fitch, had treated him for syphilis—despite a big bubo on his thigh.

In the weeks that followed, more victims surfaced: a young restaurant worker, an aged cigar maker, a housewife, a cook, another newspaper man, and a blind woman who had never left her apartment. She was case number 71.

The little morgue and lab was strained. Carbolic acid—part of the morgue and lab's daily disinfection bath—stained its floor the hue of tobacco juice around a spittoon. The building had no rugs and only a single heating grate to dispel the penetrating fog that flowed off the bay. The daily workload increased: collecting the dead, conducting autopsies, taking blood and tissue samples, growing cultures of bacteria, and injecting test animals to confirm a diagnosis. With each new death, the process began again. The small lab staff fell behind. White asked for an extra $25 a month for help in making cultures. Surgeon General Wyman vetoed the plan as too costly.

While the shell game of people moved around San Francisco Bay continued, White learned that someone had paid $100—about two months' wages—to smuggle a sick teenage boy out of San Francisco to Oakland's Chinatown. There, three days later, the boy died and a cook fell mortally ill with plague.[19] By September 1902, the toll reached eighty cases.

The Chinese government installed a new consul general in San Francisco. The new consul tried again to ban autopsies in Chinatown as a racist practice. The public health doctors refused, ruling that the victim of any suspicious death—irrespective of race—had to undergo a postmortem examination to rule out the possibility of plague. Amid this changing of the guard, the Chinatown gangsters known as "highbinders" grew bolder. Highbinders, named for their habit of coiling their queues high up under their hats, had long waged turf battles for control of lucrative Chinatown rackets.

But now the highbinders took aim at a new target: the interpreter Wong Chung. Where the state health board had seen Wong Chung's work as troublesome, some Chinese now saw it as treason. The knives were out.

"The Chinese are threatening Wong Chung because he is assisting the Marine Hospital Service in the work of eradicating plague," Mark White wired the surgeon general. ". . . Wong has been advised by friends to guard against highbinders. The situation [is] serious."[20]

One night, Wong attended a special meeting of his old colleagues at the Chinese Six Companies. As the elders talked business, several highbinders emerged from the crowd. They lunged for Wong Chung. Wong, although deceptively soft and middle-aged, was nimble. He dodged and evaded their grasp, his queue flying. The Chinese Six Companies president threw himself between Wong and his pursuers. In the scuffle, the assailants fled, disappearing into the night streets of Chinatown.[21]

After the botched assault, U.S. secretary of state John Hay moved in to shield Wong from violence. Hay formally asked the Chinese minister in Washington to help stop the harassment of "Federal Chinese employees in their official duties."[22] Under the cloak of state department protection, Wong Chung continued his medical rounds unmolested.

"Send Blue ASAP"

THE AUTUMN OF 1902 saw California's plague stalemate become a national scandal that the state could no longer conceal or deny.

In San Francisco, another white patient caught doctors off guard. Arthur Caswell, thirty-three years old, was a hard-drinking salesman at the Adolph Schwartz apparel store on 3rd Street. Caswell spent his days peddling suits, his nights hoisting glasses at a saloon. On Friday, October 24, he worked all day fitting suits on soldiers who had just shipped home from Spanish-American War duty in Manila. That night, he crawled home exhausted. On Saturday, a wave of nausea hit him harder than any hangover ever had. By Sunday morning, Caswell awoke to find a hard red lump and a gnawing pain in his groin.

He rushed to Clara Barton Hospital on Geary Boulevard. Doctors found the tender bulge in his pelvis and diagnosed Caswell with a strangulated hernia, a dangerous condition that occurs when a loop of intestine pokes through the muscle wall and becomes choked off from its blood supply. After scrubbing for emergency surgery, the surgeon made an incision in Caswell's right groin. He was shocked to find no hernia at all. Instead, he saw a skein of infected lymph glands.

The surgeon bundled Caswell into an ambulance and transferred him to the City and County Hospital. Mark White met the patient there. He examined the infected glands, which were starting to hemorrhage. There was little doubt about the cause. White injected him with Yersin's plague antiserum, and Caswell hung on.

While Caswell was fighting for his life, the leaders of the State and Provincial Health Boards of North America were fighting to get the facts about San Francisco's plague. As they gathered for their annual conference in New Haven, Connecticut, members had read dispatches from San Francisco in the New York newspapers. News of the unchecked epidemic, which ran counter to official state denials, infuriated the conferees. They moved plague to the top of their agenda and immediately passed a resolution condemning California. The plague was "a matter of grave national concern," they declared, branding the state's inaction an "irretrievable disgrace."[1]

The San Francisco Board of Supervisors monitored the meeting with trepidation. The board sent frantic appeals to Governor Gage's ranch in Downey, where the lame duck governor had gone in the waning days of his administration. They implored Gage to come to the city and acknowledge the outbreak. Gage refused.

Arthur Caswell failed to respond to the injections of antiserum. He died on Halloween, the city's eighty-ninth case of bubonic plague.

Mark White had no idea how Caswell contracted plague. He lived and worked far from Chinatown and denied visiting there in more than a year. On the plague death list, doctors wrote a footnote labeling Caswell "a rounder," as if his drinking sprees explained his fate.[2]

While Mark White struggled against rising plague and obdurate politics, Surgeon General Wyman quietly hedged his bets. He dispatched another doctor, Arthur Glennan, out West. Glennan's job was to investigate sporadic plague cases in outlying areas of California and to make one last bid for cooperation from the outgoing governor.

Glennan took the train into Southern California. In the fragrant heat of his orange and walnut groves, Gage heartily welcomed Glennan. But when he learned the nature of Glennan's mission, Gage exploded.

"That God-damned plague again!" he said.[3]

"The surgeon general only wants to clear up suspicious reports . . . without any publicity," Glennan soothed. He added he didn't want to find plague, only to find out the truth and to suggest quiet remedies.

"I'll cooperate with Surgeon General Wyman and with you, but damn the others," said Gage. "Kinyoun would have been mobbed and hanged in San Francisco if I had not prevented it," he added. "And now, I am sorry that I did."

Gage still blamed his political downfall on Kinyoun and the plague, but promised to cooperate this time if Glennan could prevent an embargo against the state. Glennan, green but cocky, thought he could do business with this governor. After all, wasn't he the surgeon general's new favorite and chosen successor to Mark White?

The race for the California governorship hurtled into its final days, with the Republicans' new nominee, Dr. George C. Pardee, favored to win. Pardee was the federal doctors' best hope, since as a physician he might take plague seriously. But to their dismay, Pardee kept silent on the subject of plague throughout his campaign.[4]

On Election Day, November 4, as San Franciscans lined up to cast their ballots, an urgent meeting convened under the dome of City Hall. U.S. Senator Perkins, who helped arrange the pact of silence about the plague, now acknowledged it openly.

"I know Surgeon General Wyman well," the senator said. "I can tell you that unless the Governor and the state health authorities recognize the existence of plague here and take steps to eradicate it, the State will be quarantined."

Governor Gage's emissary, Dr. Mathews, argued, "The disease is not bubonic plague. Every Chinaman on the West Coast has swollen glands."[5] But it was the last gasp of the Gage era. At that moment, voters were casting ballots for George Pardee. Despite his silence on the campaign trail, Pardee sent private signals to the federal doctors that he would support their fight to wipe out plague. Pardee became the public health service's best hope.

With the election over and Thanksgiving approaching, the city of San Francisco finally dealt with the rat population. It was a full year after Rupert Blue probed the death of the laundress Marguerete Saggau and concluded that her home's proximity to Chinatown was "a distance easily covered by rats in their migration."

Now, at last, the city began laying traps in earnest. Daily rounds yielded a crop of animals for the federal laboratory on Merchant Street to analyze. In Fish Alley, one of Chinatown's poorest side streets, they found a grizzled rat corpse with plague bacteria in its heart. Dead rats under a sink on Merchant Street, a few doors down from the federal lab, were infected.

In two weeks, teams harvested sixteen plague-infected rats from traps in streets and sewers. Mark White readied himself for this new phase of the campaign. To his shock, he learned he would play no role in it. On December 12, Surgeon General Wyman transferred White to Portland. San Francisco was placed under the command of the newcomer Glennan. White protested that Glennan had undermined his authority by agreeing to let Gage send detectives to spy on White—a fellow officer. It was an outrage. But Wyman didn't heed the complaint. White was out the revolving door.

Glennan soon learned it was he who had been double-crossed. The *Call* ran a story declaring that Glennan had disproven the existence of plague and had diagnosed the germ as chicken cholera. Appalled, Glennan denounced the story as fraudulent—but the damage had been done.[6]

Surgeon General Wyman now decided to visit San Francisco to view the outbreak for himself and to pay a courtesy call on outgoing Governor Gage. Then he visited the federal morgue and lab on Merchant Street. Wyman toured Chinatown—first with the governor's men and then with his own officers. He peered into plague houses, inhaling the stench of death his men breathed daily. After six days' immersion, Wyman finally felt his men's frustration and saw how politics had hamstrung their work.[7]

But to other state health leaders, the surgeon general continued to play down the threat. Writing to the health chief of Louisiana, he struck a casual and reassuring tone.

"The infection appears to be limited to Chinatown in San Francisco and to be restricted even within the limits of that locality to a very small area," Gage wrote. "I was informed by the president of the City Board of Health, Dr. Williamson, that in his opinion there was very little of it."[8]

Wyman's letter contradicted the very facts discovered by his own men. For by now, every block of Chinatown was involved in the outbreak. At least half a dozen white people had fallen victim to plague. Odd cases were cropping up in distant corners of San Francisco. Sporadic cases in Oakland were even harder to explain.

Glennan traveled to Sacramento to meet the newly elected governor, George Pardee. When he arrived at the domed white capitol, he recounted how official denial had hamstrung the public health service for three years, and he asked the new governor's help. Pardee was sympathetic, but he had his own worries. His margin of victory was thin. Open acknowledgment of plague would, he feared, anger his supporters and undermine his administration. He preferred to lend his support behind the scenes.

Glennan's confidence began to waver. Mired in the fogbank of California politics, he finally saw the impossibility of a frontal assault on the plague. As long as elected officials refused to say the word, doctors were helpless to engage the public's support. It was, he told the surgeon general, "the most complicated situation I have ever known."[9]

In January 1903, state health chiefs convened at the Willard Hotel in Washington, D.C. They were even more irate than they had been in New Haven. Once again, they censured California for its gross neglect and Governor Gage for denial that imperiled the country at large.[10]

Radicals among the state health chiefs wanted to do more than censure; they wanted to quarantine California. They also wanted the secretary of war to move the military's Pacific Coast transit service out of San Francisco. San Francisco long had feared losing military business to its rival Seattle. A quarantine and military pullout would cost San Francisco untold millions. The moderate state health chiefs just managed to defeat the measures—for the time being.

But California's delegate to the conference cautioned that the reprieve wouldn't last. Matthew Gardner, longtime physician of the Southern Pacific Railroad Co., wired his colleagues that the state now had no choice but to tell the truth. An admission, and a plan of action, were the only way to prevent a nationwide embargo.

Surgeon General Walter Wyman, who had also attended the stormy sessions, wired Arthur Glennan to confirm that the states were in earnest. Any further stalling by California would ensure a financial debacle. More important, California's denial had to end because it had become an acute embarrassment. The public health service looked weak and ineffectual after a failed three-year effort to wipe out the bubonic plague that the state still called a fake.

It was time to bring back a veteran. One federal colleague knew his way around the city, and that was Rupert Blue. But Blue was 2,200 miles away, patrolling the lakefront in Milwaukee.

Wyman wired Glennan a list of instructions and added: "Unless you wire me not needed will send Blue."[11]

Glennan, less than two months into this thankless assignment, didn't hesitate. He wired the surgeon general: "Please send Blue as soon as possible."[12]

The Perimeter Widens

"I LEAVE TOMORROW for San Francisco."[1]

Rupert Blue jotted the note to his sister Kate from Milwaukee on January 31, 1903, as he packed to leave town. He was clearing out and shipping home to South Carolina all the clothes, books, and assorted truck from his marriage that a roving sanitarian didn't need in resuming the single life out of a suitcase. Nearly thirty-five, he was starting over.

His train reached San Francisco in February—the month when the rainy season cloaked gay Victorian facades in dour gray and unleashed rivulets of mud down the cobblestones. He checked into the marble-clad Occidental Hotel on Sutter Street. Since Blue last set foot in the city, things had deteriorated. Plague's toll had almost doubled to ninety-three cases. California's negligence had made the state a national pariah. Now, as the infection seeped south of the border, its unpopularity spread. Mexico blamed a plague outbreak in Mazatlán on rats in vegetable crates from San Francisco. Ecuador barred all vessels from the state of California.

To prevent a revolt by other states and countries, Glennan told California it must acknowledge the plague and adopt a plan to wipe it out. Businessmen hedged around uneasily, drafting a weasel-worded statement about California's "alleged plague." Glennan got angry. Speak plainly, he said, or face ruin. He drafted a declaration, which the businessmen reluctantly signed. Then together they marched to City Hall to confront the mayor.

Mayor Schmitz, outnumbered, couldn't charm his way out. With Glennan and the businessmen looking on, the mayor grimly scratched his signature. Then Glennan, triumphant, boarded a train for Sacramento to get the governor's signature. Governor Pardee, while he'd never denied the plague, wasn't eager to trumpet it to the world, either. But he, too, had no choice. With Schmitz and Pardee inking the deal, and Blue back in town to manage the Chinatown cleanup, Glennan told the surgeon general the situation was under control.[2]

Blue's first task was managing a joint plan of action to clean up plague houses and clear out rat refuges. The crux of the plan was this: The state would hire three medical inspectors, two sanitary engineers, and two Chinese interpreters. The city would lay traps and poison bait for rats. Chinatown streets would be washed regularly. Dupont Street would get a coat of asphalt. The public health service would inspect the sick and the dead, run the plague lab, and report to Washington on the cleanup and the caseload.

Blue was confident. "Thing are smoothly moving," he jotted in the plague lab journal.[3] But that season, his public health officers landed in the infirmary. Drs. Glennan, Currie, and Lloyd all came down with influenza. Their stenographer landed in the pesthouse with smallpox. Their second Chinese interpreter, Fong Dont, got measles. Only Blue stayed on his feet.

He had to. Warm weather would soon bring out the fleas in droves. Chinatown's cleanup went into high gear with a frenzy of cleansing, exterminating, and remodeling. The smoking and scrubbing out of germs continued. Workers lugged hand pumps into buildings, spraying a mist of carbolic acid that left a musty scent of mothballs. They stirred smoking pots of sulfur, casting a fog that reeked of rotten eggs. And they sprinkled chlorinated lime in houses, releasing a vapor of chlorine gas that drove the residents outside, gasping for air. To many Chinese, the treatment seemed like harassment at best, poisoning at worst.

Next Blue undertook his assault on rats. To be successful, he had to appeal to their palates. Blue knew rats were gourmets—they would never take boring bait—so he devised a varied menu, including cheese in a Welsh rabbit and rye bread sandwiches with bacon. He spiked the meals with arsenic or phosphorous poison.

A third front of the war was aimed at the very structure of Chinatown. Over the years, a racially biased housing market had sealed the growing population into the narrow district. Apartments had sprouted ramshackle additions to stretch crowded living space. Wooden porches and balconies, tacked on to buildings, now overhung the streets, leaving the ground below dark and damp under a layer of trash. Blue asked the city board of health to declare the additions unsanitary and schedule them for demolition.

The Chinese protested that the demolitions were unfair. Haphazard extensions were necessary to stretch the overcrowded living space. They weren't to blame for the overcrowding, they said. They were simply caught in the squeeze.

Landlords sued to block the demolitions. Court injunctions halted the work. Glennan and Blue attended public hearings at the board of health, arguing that porches and balconies were a health nuisance. The campaign was unpopular, but the alternative was even worse: a proposal by white merchants suggested that the city clear the Chinese and relocate them to Hunter's Point.[4] Blue's program, while tough, at least had the virtue of trying to make Chinatown more habitable.

Finally, sanitary engineers got a green light to begin prying the rotten balconies off Chinatown apartments. Stacks of splintered timber grew in the street.

The woodpiles drew the eyes of poor scavengers.

One sharp-eyed passerby was a Sicilian railroad man named Pietro Spadafora. With his wife, two children, and aged mother, Spadafora lived on an alley in the city's Latin Quarter, just a few blocks north of Chinatown. Each day, he crossed Chinatown on his way to and from work at the Southern Pacific Railroad yards south of Market Street. Evenings after work, he paused in Chinatown to hunt for bargains among the sidewalk bins of cabbages and bitter greens, oranges and onions. One night he saw an even better bargain: free firewood. Surely a poor man could be forgiven if he took an armload to light his stove and chase the chill of a foggy summer night.

Pietro mounted the steps to his Victorian row house at 19 Jasper Place and presented his family with the makings of dinner and a good fire. A couple of days after this repast, Pietro fell ill. His forehead burned, his muscles ached, his stomach revolted, and all the strength fled from his limbs. Too weak to protest, he was carted off to the Southern Pacific Hospital, his company's infirmary, on Mission Street.

Shortly after they took her son, Pietro's mother found a tender lump low in her belly. Her fever rose. She burned and shivered by turns. Still, she did not go to the hospital but remained at home, awaiting her son's return.

Pietro did not come home. He died on July 19 in the Southern Pacific Hospital, leaving his widow with two small children. When doctors rushed to the house on Jasper Place to investigate, they found his mother, Pietra Brancato, slipping from consciousness into coma. Mrs. Brancato survived her son by little more than a day. Both were victims of bubonic plague.

Blue ruminated about the source of this case, twisting his mustache. Compared to the tenements of Chinatown, a few blocks to the south, the houses in the Latin Quarter were new, spacious, and sound. Next, he pondered Pietro's travels about town. On his rounds from North Beach to his job in the district south of Market Street, he shopped in Chinatown, but plague seemed unlikely to lurk in his grocery basket. Then there was the matter of the debris.

The rotten timber, discarded from condemned buildings, was being stolen for firewood. After wrestling with the peculiar facts of the case, Blue could only conclude that Pietro Spadafora had carried home kindling from a plague house that was crawling with fleas. For warming his hearth with pilfered wood, he and his mother paid with their lives.[5]

Suddenly, Blue worried that other scavengers might carry plague-infested wood into other homes. So he quickly ordered that all debris from condemned dwellings be dredged with powdered lime—a disinfectant that rendered it unusable as firewood. The debris would then be guarded by police until it could be safely burned, beyond the reach of poor pilferers. Finally, he ordered inspectors to press northward into the flats and row houses of the bustling Latin Quarter.

In the summer of 1903, when Arthur Glennan was recalled to Washington for a new assignment, Blue finally took formal command of the San Francisco plague operation. It was the function he'd fulfilled for some time, the role he was destined to play. Despite Glennan's political naïveté and tactical missteps, Blue was a gracious successor. He credited his predecessor for working to unite the city's warring factions, and he vowed to finish the job.

Under Blue's direction, the rat trapping and cleanup of Chinatown became more systematic. Each week, he filed reports on the number of dwellings inspected and condemned, the number of rats trapped and autopsied, the number of people visited, both sick and dead. As a part of this grisly accounting, Surgeon General Wyman asked to know the race of each victim. It was a desperate but misguided search for clues, since plague was starting to defy racial theories of susceptibility.

With the death of Pietro Spadafora and his mother, Blue's team began inspecting thousands of white apartments in the cosmopolitan Latin Quarter. For the first time, Caucasian homes outnumbered those of Chinese on the inspection log.

All hope of containing plague in one geographic area evaporated. Another quarter was now infected, Blue told the surgeon general. Gone, too, was the logic of assessing risk by nationality. The Latin Quarter, now called North Beach, was home to Portuguese, Mexican, Italian, and French households. A melting pot of races, it now turned into a crucible of risk. The perimeter was widening.[6]

The Chamber of Commerce, unimpressed with moves to make Chinatown more livable, resumed the cry to raze the district outright. "Chinatown menaces every man and every family and every interest in San Francisco, and sooner or later it must be wiped out," the chamber declared. "No amount of cleansing and scouring will give us permanent relief."[7]

But health was just a pretext. The fact was that Chinatown sat on prime land, surrounded by Union Square, Nob Hill, and the financial district. Businessmen wanted to relocate the Chinese people to a spot where a quarantine wouldn't interrupt downtown businesses. Blue still hoped to make Chinatown healthy.

One day Blue looked up from his labors and was surprised to find his old University of Virginia friend and sometime competitor, Joe Guthrie. They celebrated their reunion like college boys. Touring the San Francisco night spots, they painted the town red. "This we did to the Queen's taste," he wrote Kate, "managing however to keep out of the hands of the police. . . ."[8]

After his night out, Blue must have realized how thoroughly he'd submerged his personal into his professional life since his split with Juliette. During his marriage, his letters were loquacious and charming, filled with wordplay and sketches of the people and places he encountered. Afterward, they were brief, telegraphic, and guarded. Kate, for her part, avoided references to her brother's doomed marriage. But now Blue lowered his emotional drawbridge, reaching out for more family contact. "Dear child," he teased her, "don't count letters with me, but write often." And he closed, "With dearest love to all, Yours, Rupert."

Soon enough, it was back to work. Ignoring Chamber of Commerce calls to destroy and relocate Chinatown, Blue pushed deeper into the very foundations of the district. He wanted to replace the porous wooden cellars that served as rat catacombs with hardened, rat-proof concrete basements. He would clear trash-choked cellars and courtyards, scrape away a foot of subsoil, and pour cement floors. He dubbed this phase of the work "building out the plague."

With cases in Chinatown slowing to a handful, Blue couldn't suppress his feelings of progress. But the steady pulse of plague cases left him uneasy.

In the case of a fifty-four-year-old actor named Chin Lai, it was the doctors who beheld his final breathtaking performance. While declaiming his lines in a historical drama, Chin was hit by a wave of vertigo, fever, and chills. His friends hastily moved Chin from the theater to a quarantine house on Fish Alley. Federal doctors making a house call were dumbfounded: There sat the actor, robust and animated, talking to doctors until one hour before his death. In a bravura turn, he seemed to defy infection in his glands and bloodstream until a wave of sepsis overwhelmed him. Then he sank swiftly, and the light left his eyes.

Occasionally, the coffin shops got orders for very small boxes. Jew Sue and Slick Chat were seven-year-old girls who lived and played one block apart on Washington Street. The little girls abandoned their sidewalk games and took to bed with fevers almost simultaneously. Surely they would recover. So no one called the federal doctors to come and check the girls until they died, just three days apart on November 4 and 7.

Down at City Hall, Eugene Schmitz and Abe Ruef, though increasingly bold in their graft, swept to easy reelection in November 1903. Not everyone was happy with the incumbents. A crusading newspaper editor Fremont Older of the *Bulletin* launched a campaign of muckraking. He published a cartoon captioned "Our Mayor" depicting not Schmitz, but his counselor Ruef on a throne, surrounded by bags of gold, smoking a fat cigar. But muckrakers couldn't put a dent in their popularity. Many San Franciscans thought the cartoon unfair: Everybody knew Ruef didn't smoke.[9]

Blue brooded and searched his soul about gaps in the plague campaign. He decided that the rat-killing operation was not aggressive enough. He now proposed a bold expansion of the rodent slaughter, one that would cover the whole of San Francisco. Moreover, Blue wanted to offer an incentive to the rat catchers, borrowing a strategy from the sheriffs of the Old West. He would offer citizens a bounty for bringing in rats—dead or alive.[10]

First, official rat trappers would be paid a bonus of 10 cents in addition to their daily wage for every rat they delivered. The program ran a calculated risk. There was a danger that poor desperadoes might import rodents for the cash, introducing even more vermin into the rat-ridden city. But the need was so great that the bounty program was eventually expanded to include all citizens, and the reward was raised to two and even four bits.

Blue decided to be pragmatic about coaxing support from the newspapers. Without mentioning plague, he asked their support for rat eradication on the grounds of city hygiene. The *Chronicle*—unclear that the goal was to get rid of rodents—came back with a quixotic counterproposal. Why not unleash ferrets as rat catchers?

IN NOVEMBER, CLOUDBURSTS SWEPT off the Pacific, quenching the long dry season. Seasoned plague fighters knew the cold would force vermin back underground, bringing a deceptive pause in human cases. But, Blue warned his colleagues, the germs were hibernating, and this was only an intermission.

Still, by New Year's 1904, the normally cautious Blue felt a surge of optimism. Chinatown's health was looking up. He dared to hope that the outbreak might burn itself out. Success seemed within his reach, if not yet in his grasp.

The city was visibly cleaner. It was also bigger and brassier. The population now topped the four hundred thousand mark. Merchants wired Geary Street with electricity, blazing a light trail in the night labyrinth of the city. The Anti-Saloon League took a dim view of all this, warning that Frisco after dark was "Satan's seat, sodden with saloons and sated with liquefied sin."[11]

Of course, sin drew as many tourists as sunshine, as Blue well knew, having tasted its nightlife.

Just then, a flurry of small earthquakes shook Northern California. It wasn't enough to do any damage, but it seemed like a premonition. The *Sacramento Bee*'s page one headline mocked the inevitability of a seismic catastrophe:

"YOU, YOU I WANT," SAID THE EARTHQUAKE.
"NOT YET," SAID SAN FRANCISCO.[12]

At City Hall, Mayor Schmitz finally won the right to install his own city board of health. The old "bubonic board" was out; the new board immediately started cutting the Chinatown cleanup staff. Schmitz wanted the federal doctors to stop work and clear out of town.

To win back City Hall's fickle support, Blue deployed a charm offensive. He marched down to the board of supervisors, who held the purse strings. He pointed to the visible transformation of Chinatown: The rickety balconies and porches were gone, the buildings had new concrete foundations, and leaky old sewer pipes were repaired—even the air was fresher.

Let us keep trapping rats. Let us keep inspecting the sick and the dead. Let us keep working until the city is restored to health, he implored them. Whether it was because of his logic or his courtly manners, Blue won a reprieve.

Three silent witnesses in January proved the battle wasn't over: A cucumber farmer, an elderly man on Fish Alley, and a housewife on Jackson Street all died. The woman, twenty-six-year-old Ho Mon Chin Shee, collapsed with a fever of 108.5—the highest recorded since the outbreak.

"The appearance at this time of three suspicious cases was a surprise and a matter of regret," Blue said. "I presume they are the result of the dry weather we have had since December 21st." The weather was only an excuse; the city was still infected.[13]

The solution lay underground. This trio of cases clustered around the intersection of Jackson and Fish Alley, near the Jackson Street Theatre. Blue sent inspectors out to poke around. Searching the underground pipes, they traced the probable infection source to a broken sewer pipe harboring vermin under the theater. Workers patched the pipe, doused the buildings with bichloride of mercury, then sprinkled them with lime. They also gutted the wooden basements and poured a concrete rat barrier.

The gritty work ground on door-to-door. In the week ending January 9, the health officers inspected 1,916 rooms. They checked 1,998 people. They limed and disinfected 967 sites around Chinatown. Week in, week out, they took temperatures, felt glands, scrubbed houses, and cemented cellars. It was sidewalk sanitation as much as it was medicine.

The board of supervisors' finance committee now put the Washington doctors on month-to-month funding. Blue attended the supervisors' meetings, hoping for more but willing to economize. His bigger fear was that City Hall would revert to the old practice of denying plague. To arouse public awareness and support, he needed City Hall to admit the truth, or at least to not lie about it.

But if the politicians unsettled his hopes in January, a cluster of new cases would all but shatter them in February.

The Seamstresses

KATIE CUKA WAS AN eighteen-year-old Ohio native who came to San Francisco and ended up working as a seamstress. At the S. N. Wood Company clothing factory on Geary Boulevard, she helped turn bolts of tweed woolens into $10 men's suits. While working one afternoon, she complained of a chill. Suddenly she felt woozy; her head spun, and then everything went black.

Following her fainting spell, Katie was rushed to the city's French Hospital, where doctors found she had a high fever and swollen glands. After drawing fluid from her lymph glands, they recoiled to find it brimming with suspicious bacteria. The significance didn't escape them. In a panic, the doctors sent Katie home to her lodgings on Natoma Street, south of the Market Street slot. The city health department, tipped off about the possible plague case, sent a horse-drawn ambulance to bring her to the City and County Hospital's isolation cottage.

Federal doctors swooped down on the suit factory with questions. Were there any more seamstresses who were ill?

The foreman said he had two more girls on the sick list. Mary Fremont, a girl living near Katie, turned out to have a simple sore throat. But Irene Rossi, daughter of an Italian peddler, was down with a fever in the Latin Quarter. The doctors went to investigate.

When they arrived at the Rossi row house on Varennes Street,[1] they saw that they were too late. They found the stricken family in black, planning Irene's funeral. Their eighteen-year-old had gone downhill rapidly; from a fever, chills, pounding head, and aching chest, she had progressed to racking coughs that brought up streaks of blood, then a foamy fluid that looked like raspberry syrup. Pneumonia, they called it. As her parents hovered helplessly, she had died gasping. During their vigil, the Rossis bent close, inhaling the same air, until their prayers expired with her.

Bowed by grief, Luisa and Giuseppe Rossi raised haunted eyes from the waxen face of their child to the doctors, who no doubt felt stricken as they paused on the threshold, absorbing the awful scene. After murmuring condolences, the doctors asked permission to perform an autopsy.

Torn by grief, his eyes blazing darkly, Giuseppe Rossi said no. The doctors pressed gently, saying it was required for all suspicious sickness. Only if the autopsy took place that night, Rossi said, so that Irene could be buried the next day as planned. And only, he added, if he could accompany her to the morgue. The doctors had no choice.

Late that night, just outside the circle of lamplight, Giuseppe Rossi witnessed what no father should ever see: doctors making the long incision, cutting the snips of tissue from his daughter, preserving them in glass like relics of the saints.

Giuseppe's frenzied mourning, his burning gaze, masked something more—something the doctors had missed. Later, Blue would recognize that the bereaved father was so "buoyed up by grief or excitement" that no one—least of all the father himself—recognized that he too was falling sick.[2] But the day after the funeral, the fifty-four-year-old peddler collapsed, not from grief but from fever. Soon he was coughing blood as his daughter had. By February 12, four days after his daughter, Giuseppe Rossi himself lay dead.

Seventeen doctors crowded around the autopsy table, Rupert Blue among them. The incision parted skin, muscle, and bone to reveal the lungs, the bellows of the body that are normally a rich wine red with oxygen but were now clotted with the germs that killed father and daughter.

The autopsies of both found the cause of death to be pneumonic plague. Explosively contagious, it would have imperiled anyone who had visited the coughing girl in her sickroom and breathed its germ-laden air. Luisa Rossi, the girl's mother, was in the most danger, but before she could be placed in isolation, she vanished. Health officers searched the Latin Quarter for her, to no avail. Finally, a doctor's tip led them to the Richmond district out on the city's western edge. There, they found Mrs. Rossi, who had taken refuge from her grief at her brother's home on Lake Street and 13th Avenue. She was already burning with fever.

On February 17, the forty-five-year-old Mrs. Rossi followed her daughter and husband into death. At her autopsy, Blue and Currie saw her lungs congealed with pockets of infection. Pneumonic plague, again, was the diagnosis. That same day, Mrs. Rossi's brother Joseph fell sick, with tender and swollen glands in his groin and armpit. The symptoms looked suspicious. But Joseph refused to let doctors pierce his glands to obtain a fluid sample.

Doctors reasoned, then argued, but they failed to persuade him. They fumed and swallowed their frustration. Joseph Rossi appeared to have a mild case of bubonic plague. But his was a case that would have to remain unconfirmed—a gap in the puzzle.

"Please send 200 bottles fresh Yersin," Blue wired urgently to Washington.[3] He would need that much plague antiserum and more if this cluster grew. Wyman shipped 150 bottles, and Blue ordered 50 more from Sharp & Dohme Chemists in New York City. Doctors canvassed the Latin Quarter for anyone who might have been exposed. Joseph Rossi stubbornly stood by his refusal to allow a biopsy. But hedging his bets, he agreed to take injections of the antiserum.

Sanitation workers engulfed the row house at 6 Varennes Street with sulfur fumigation, bichloride of mercury solution, and sprinklings of lime. They built a pyre in the street and burned the linens from the sickroom beds. Where the three Rossis once lived, only a rank ghost of sulfur and veil of chemicals hung suspended in the air.

Meanwhile, the factory girl Katie Cuka held her grip on life at the county hospital. The young seamstress would survive her ordeal. So would Joseph Rossi. But where the factory girls first became infected—at home or at work—was anyone's guess. Neither site was anywhere near Chinatown. Once again, plague rats were outflanking the doctors with a pattern no one could explain.

After a harrowing two weeks, Blue could breathe again. Finally he felt confident enough to declare the cluster contained. "I believe," he wrote the surgeon general on February 23, "we have seen the last of the pneumonic cases to be expected from the infection at No. 6 [Varennes] Street in the Rossi family."[4]

Word that a white family was wiped out by plague raced through the medical community. For the first time, people felt a threat in their midst. Doctors telephoned Blue, anxiously asking about the availability of supplies of the antiserum. Along with a new sense of vulnerability, a new candor was born. For the first time, community physicians reluctantly admitted that they had seen such cases before.

"I am unable to decide whether these recent cases among the whites represent an increase, or whether they are the result of a desire on the part of physicians to openly diagnose plague," Blue told Wyman. "It would appear from conversations we have had with some of them, that they have had such cases before, but were not willing to make the diagnosis."[5]

The city was now in its fifth year of a smoldering plague. Blue must have felt outraged that doctors were only now acknowledging the outbreak. But whatever his frustration, he had to master it. He couldn't afford the indulgence of an outburst. He had to keep these doctors on his side. Besides, it was too late to backtrack or to count the innumerable dead. He could only move on.

Blue focused instead on uniting the factions of the city into a fragile coalition. He invited state and local health officials to meet with businessmen and federal doctors at the Merchant Street lab. He opened the floor to any issue—from how to fund the plague campaign to how to curb spitting on the sidewalk. Calling itself the Public Health Commission of California, the group even elected Rupert Blue as its president. After years of struggle, Blue was surprised to find he had actually become popular.

Blue's extermination drive was now getting impressive results with the Danysz rat virus sold by the Pasteur Institute. In reality, it was simply *Bacillus typhimurium*, a bug related to a common food poisoning bacterium. Mixed with yellow cornmeal, the poison was spread through dwellings, stores, houses, and basements. The Chinese were dubious at first, but when they saw that it didn't hurt humans or domestic animals, they reluctantly accepted it. When they saw that it worked, they even asked for it. The product yielded a bumper crop of dead rats.

By late May, optimism surged again. Almost one hundred days

had passed since the last plague cases. It was the longest intermission since the outbreak began in March 1900. Blue told Wyman he hoped the mayor would stay friendly and keep funding his plan to gird rat-proof foundations throughout all of Chinatown by the year's end.

The city was looking better. The retreat of plague and the pristine state of Chinatown was now a potent lure for speculators. Property values surged. The district looked so good, merchants proposed to sell $10 million in bonds and turn Chinatown into parkland. To Blue's disgust, a group of doctors formed an investment company to buy up Chinatown property. "The company was not formed for the purpose of obtaining better sanitary conditions for San Francisco," he wrote indignantly to Washington, "but merely for money-making."[6] Uncharacteristically, the city rejected the scheme.

As word of the city's progress spread, the plague pioneer Shibasaburo Kitasato, who had raced Alexandre Yersin to identify the bacterium, now sent his assistant from Japan to San Francisco to study Blue's methods. The Japanese visitor mainly wanted to study Blue's strategy of "building out the plague." Blue gave him a tour, proudly noting that the visitor scribbled copious notes about "everything that was in sight."[7]

Surprisingly, the cleanup seemed to be slashing rates of sickness overall. "There has been a remarkable decrease in the death rate for the past year, 388 as compared to 464 of the preceding year," Blue rejoiced. He hoped to persuade the most hardened skeptics in Chinatown to join forces with him. "Even the Chinese should be able to reason out the cause," he wrote Washington, "and join us in greater endeavors than before."[8]

When six months elapsed following the Rossi deaths, city fathers started agitating for a clean bill of health for San Francisco. "The long interval that has occurred is considered by some of the people here to warrant the claim of extirpation of the disease," said a wary Blue. But he added, "If by the beginning of the rainy season no case has occurred, then we may speak more confidently of eradication."[9]

Furnishing ammunition for city exterminators, Blue's laboratory on Merchant Street was now brewing up batches of Danysz rat poison in quantity. He needed enough to bait Chinatown, the Japanese district, and the Latin Quarter. That winter, however, the laboratory, with its lone heating grate, was so cold that the cultures of *B. ty-*

phimurium refused to grow. With a little dime-store ingenuity, his men wrapped hot-water bottles around the bouillon cultures, and the bugs multiplied like mad.[10]

Blue sent New Year's wishes to Surgeon General Wyman and recommended continuing inspections well into 1905 as insurance that the eradication was complete. The city had other ideas. San Francisco was eager to wrap up the plague campaign. Chinatown was clean and more rat-free than most of the city. Despite his conservatism, Blue had to admit that the epidemic's retreat had held firm for eleven months. It was probably safe to wind down the operation.

San Francisco didn't evict Blue as unceremoniously as it had his predecessor Joseph Kinyoun. Indeed, just after the rainy Valentine's Day of 1905, the city health department sent him a municipal valentine, expressing "our thanks . . . to Dr. Rupert Blue for his skillful and energetic co-operation in all that has pertained to the welfare of San Francisco's high sanitary state and commercial prosperity."[11]

After 121 cases of plague and 113 deaths, San Francisco's plague seemed over. Blue dismantled his team of inspectors, wreckers, and disinfectors. Then he handed over the keys to the Merchant Street plague lab to Donald Currie, who would close the shop.

But Blue couldn't forget the unsolved cases. Despite his success in Chinatown, he was nagged by a sense of unfinished business. There was the case of Charles Bock, a twenty-nine-year-old blacksmith from the East Bay village of Pacheco. Troubled by fever and a leaden ache in his chest, Bock was ferried to San Francisco by his brother. During the arduous day-long trip, the blacksmith's condition deteriorated. One hour after being admitted to German Hospital, he was dead. His spleen, glands, and chest muscles were riddled with plague.

Bock hadn't visited the city for a month prior to his death. That meant he must have become infected near his home, but how? Although just a few miles away from foggy San Francisco, the East Bay was a different world: a sun-baked terrain of tawny hills studded with oak. If you believed the conventional medical wisdom, it was a most unlikely spot for plague. Plague was a tropical disease that thrived in steamy settings. If San Francisco had once seemed too cold for plague, the East Bay seemed in turn too dry. San Francisco had abundant rats; the East Bay had few. All it had were feathery-tailed ground squirrels, and no one had any proof that squirrels played a role in the plague. But the possibility haunted Blue. Squirrels, he realized, infested the whole state.

There was no time to brood about it. For Surgeon General Wyman dispatched a terse telegram bearing new orders for Blue to transfer to Norfolk, Virginia. There, he would treat sick and injured sailors in the port city famed for its oysters. He was also in line for a job as the chief medical officer at the nearby Jamestown Exposition, marking the three hundredth anniversary of the country's first English-speaking colony. He packed up his blue dress uniform and his workaday khakis and left on April 4, 1905.

A celebration of American military might, the Jamestown Exposition was an odd mix of military hardware and western myth, naval flotillas and Wild West shows featuring mock cowboy and Indian battles. As chief of health and hygiene, Blue would be responsible for preventing disease outbreaks that might mar the event. For an epidemic fighter, it was hardly a blood-stirring challenge.

But Blue was content to be back in the South, to hear lambent southern accents, soak up the sun, and feast on the melons his brother Bill would plant that year. He felt he needed to steam the Pacific fog out of his bones in the heat of a southern summer and that he hadn't seen the sunshine since leaving Galveston in 1894. He wrote Kate: "Many times I have changed stations since then and have served in Italy, but the summer failed in all of them."[12]

A tentative thaw was beginning. For in the same letter, Blue divulged that he had ventured back into social life for the first time since his divorce. Invited to a big society wedding in Norfolk, he felt his blood stir. "The girls are very pretty and stylish withal," he confided to Kate. "Perhaps I shall meet my fate among them. You see, I have forgotten the unpleasant past." The cream of Norfolk society, he assured her, were big enough to overlook a gentleman's past—be he a divorced doctor or traveling sanitarian.

In the South, Blue could look after his family. He sent money home regularly. When Annie Maria had a bout of rheumatism, he dispensed medical advice. He searched the city for opera music to send to Henriette. "I would so delight," he wrote them, "in an evening of grand opera at home."[13] When he got wind of a spat, he counseled Kate and Henriette on how to keep peace at home. "Life at best is a burden," he lectured them, "made up largely of concessions, of denials and of the elimination of ego as much as possible in the home circle."

The year 1905 also saw Blue confirm the most enduring comradeship of his life. It had all started four years earlier when a sailor had gotten drunk, slipped on the ice, and broken his leg.

It was a frigid winter day in Milwaukee in January 1901 when the injured sailor consulted William Colby Rucker, a young doctor struggling to establish a private practice. The sailor, short on funds to pay for treatment, asked Rucker to send him to see a Dr. Rupert Blue, who worked for the federal government treating injured seamen for free. Rucker sought out Blue's boardinghouse to arrange it. He remembered being struck by the power of Blue's physical presence:

"As he came down the broad stairs to greet me, I thought I had never seen a finer looking man in all my life," Rucker recalled, "a big handsome man . . . charmingly courteous to me, and as I was a youngster of 25, I was much flattered. A nice intimacy sprang up between us."[14]

When the two doctors met again at medical society meetings, Rucker confided that he had fallen in love with a honey-haired schoolteacher and needed to launch his medical career to provide for her. Blue recommended applying for the public health service, and Rucker eagerly enlisted. He married his schoolteacher, Annette, and had a son named Colby. In 1905, Blue and Rucker were reunited when both were assigned to the Norfolk station.

Norfolk was placid after San Francisco. But farther south, the Gulf coast was under assault by *Aedes aegypti* mosquitoes. By midsummer came word that the citizens of New Orleans were falling ill with temperatures and jaundice: yellow fever.

Blue and Rucker were among the two dozen officers dispatched by Washington to fight the epidemic. They were placed under the command of Blue's old nemesis—Joseph White. The compact, lively Rucker was the perfect foil to the quiet giant Blue. Where Blue was cautious and laconic, Rucker was warm and extroverted.

In Louisiana, Blue faced down a "shotgun quarantine"—a circle of farmers who fended off the public health service by brandishing firearms at the federal doctors.[15]

Rucker's turf included New Orleans's houses of worship and

houses of ill fame. And both responded to his cocktail of charm and guile. When parishioners of one church came down with yellow fever, Rucker discovered mosquitoes breeding in the holy water. After an old priest refused to drain or salt the fonts, Rucker stealthily slipped disinfecting tablets into the vessel. When forced to fumigate the sanctuary, Rucker took the sting out of the treatment by anointing the church statues with a protective coat of petroleum jelly. The priest was happy, and his parishioners got well.

Rucker's magic with the women inside an epidemic zone was honed by his encounter with a very tough crowd: the madams of Storeyville, the city's famous red-light district. These hard-boiled businesswomen wanted no part of public health. The whores, whom Rucker found childlike and innocent, loved his visits. He issued a challenge to the madams: When your girls take sick, call me or I'll shut you down. Reluctantly they accepted his rule, capping cisterns and screening porches to bar mosquitoes.

Soon Storeyville was a model of public health. But Rucker himself began to sweat, and saw in his oddly amber skin and eyeballs the unmistakable symptoms of the virus nicknamed "yellow jack." While he languished in the infirmary, his senior officer and his patients felt his absence.

"Dr. Rucker . . . is one of our merriest officers, and those of us who are left miss him from our daily dinners and confabulations," Blue wrote to his sister Kate.[16] The Storeyville women missed him, too, bearing bouquets to his hospital bedside. On his return to rounds, the women in unison shouted a raucous "Welcome back!" from their wrought-iron balconies.[17]

Once Rucker was back at work, Rupert wrote Kate, "The suppression of the fever is simply a matter of time. We have a death grip on it and do not intend to 'leave go' until the question of supremacy is settled."[18] They got help from the weather. Yellow fever was over by the first frost of 1905. It wasn't the last time Blue and Rucker would join forces against an epidemic. But their next chance followed a cataclysm neither one could have envisioned.

Earthquake

◈

AT 5:12 A.M. ON WEDNESDAY, April 18, 1906, the ground beneath San Francisco convulsed. There was a groan of grinding mortar and a thunder of raining brick and stone. Twisting timber shrieked and snapped into splintered kindling. After forty-five seconds, the roiling paused a moment, and then a second shock wave hit, more violent than the first.[1]

From a hundred thousand fractured rooms came cries of shock and pain. Sleepers, hurled from their beds, threw coats over nightclothes, grabbed children, and poured into the street. Some yanked frantically on bedroom doors, trapped in shifting frames that no longer fit. Buildings listed drunkenly off their foundations. Wooden cottages collapsed like houses of cards, rows of flats like dominoes. Brick facades peeled off and crashed into the street, exposing what looked like a doll's house. Streetcar tracks buckled in serpentine snarls.

South of Market Street, where tracts sat precariously on landfill, the ground liquefied over ancient waterfront and wetlands. The four-story Valencia Hotel, a working-class lodging house, sank into its fluid foundation. With only its top story protruding above ground, lodgers on the lower floors were submerged and drowned.

Dozens of small fires burst from toppled chimneys and cracked stove flues. Fire alarms stayed strangely silent. The alarm center on

Brenham Place had been destroyed. At one station, fire horses bolted in fear, so firefighters had to tow their engines by hand. When they hooked up their hoses, only droplets trickled out, so the firefighters siphoned leaky sewage to spray on the flames.

Steers being herded to the Potrero stockyards were spooked by the shaking and stampeded along Mission Street. To avoid being trampled, bystanders shot the crazed cattle between the eyes.

On Merchant Street, near the federal morgue and laboratory, fish dealer Alex Paladini was unloading the morning's catch when the earthquake disintegrated buildings around him, burying horses, drivers, wagons, and fish under tons of bricks and mortar. The steeds' necks protruded from the debris, their manes caked with dust, tongues lolling. The neighborhood around the morgue was now one giant street of the dead.

The ground shock savaged City Hall. Its regal dome teetered on empty ribs. All around it stretched acres of rubble. Before the day was over, flames devoured municipal records, incinerating all city history before 1906.

Mayor Eugene Schmitz, who had been reelected despite an ongoing graft probe, now played his role with cool command. He closed the saloons. He imposed a curfew from dark until dawn. When rioters raided liquor and cigar shops, he issued an executive order for federal troops and police to shoot looters on sight. From the ruins of City Hall, he moved the seat of government to the Hall of Justice on Kearny Street, then to the Fairmont Hotel, then to a hall in the Western Addition, keeping one step ahead of the flames.

Schmitz wired the mayor of Oakland, demanding hoses and dynamite. From the capital in Sacramento, Governor George Pardee boarded a train toward the stricken city, setting up his base of operations in Oakland, where phone and wire service remained intact. He telegraphed Los Angeles, imploring: "For God's sake send food."[2]

Central Emergency Hospital collapsed, killing doctors and nurses. Its patients were moved to the Mechanics' Pavilion. The night before, the pavilion had been awhirl with roller skaters competing in a tournament. Now it was a war zone, littered with broken bodies and doctors racing about in desperate triage.

As the Palace Hotel writhed and shuddered, beds bucking and

chandeliers crashing, the tenor Enrico Caruso, fresh from singing the role of Don José in *Carmen,* was wrenched from his dreams into a nightmare. After throwing on his fur coat, the portly star ran into the street and headed north toward the St. Francis Hotel, where his opera colleagues had been staying. Some say he wept. "Hell of a place!" Caruso cried. "I never come back here." Upon his return to Italy, he kept his promise and never sang in the city again.[3]

In Hayes Valley, a woman tried to cook breakfast on a broken stove and succeeded in igniting the walls of her frame house. The resulting blaze, called the "ham and eggs fire," ate quickly through the wooden Victorian neighborhood, growing into a major conflagration. Crossing Van Ness Avenue, it torched church steeples in its path, burning on to the Civic Center, where blowing cinders lit the roof of the Mechanics' Pavilion. As smoke seeped into the makeshift hospital, doctors again evacuated patients. As afternoon turned to evening, the "ham and eggs fire" roared south and merged with a fire in the Mission district.

Two other fires coalesced into a second giant inferno. At Delmonico's restaurant, a cooking fire burned north and merged with a big blaze in the wholesale district that joined the waterfront and Chinatown. From these two infernos blossomed the Great Fire, which would rage for three days.

Fiction writers plundered their imaginations for words to describe the sight. The novelist Mary Austin wrote that the fire gave off a "lurid glow like the unearthly flush on the face of a dying man."[4] Another eyewitness to the disaster, the novelist Jack London, trod the smoking city with his wife, Charmian.

"A sickly light was creeping over the face of things," London wrote. "Once only the sun broke through the smoke-pall, blood red, and showing a quarter its usual size. The smoke-pall itself, viewed from beneath, was a rose color that pulsed and fluttered with lavender shades. Then it turned mauve and yellow and dun. There was no sun. And so dawned the second day on stricken San Francisco."[5]

Surrounded on three sides by water, the city was dry. The major water distribution mains all over the city had ruptured. As a result, fire hoses couldn't tap the eighty million gallons of water stored in city reservoirs.[6] Hugging the waterfront from Fort Mason to Hunter's Point, tugboats pumped seawater from the bay into hoses stretched ashore. The other weapon was dynamite, ignited to carve firebreaks between the walls of flame. Charges were exploded along Van Ness Avenue to halt the westward march of the Great Fire. But other explosions ignited by inexperienced hands served only to launch firebrands that spread the blazes.

A drunken munitions man, John Bermingham, carted explosives into Chinatown to demolish the wreckage and ended up starting sixty fires. As witnesses watched in horror, he lurched around setting charges that blew up buildings with people still trapped inside. Bodies flew fifty feet above the rubble, falling back into the flames below.[7]

Atrocities were rumored—of jewel thieves cutting the fingers and ears from corpses, of bloodthirsty troops bayoneting innocent citizens. As teams of rescuers clawed frantically to free the injured from rubble, some lost a race with the approaching fires. One man, hopelessly pinned down by debris, begged his rescuers to kill him before the flames burned him alive. A gunman stepped from the crowd, gravely confirmed the trapped man's last wishes, drew a pistol, and fired. He then turned himself in to the mayor, who commended his humane act.[8]

Tallying losses of such magnitude was almost impossible. In a telegram to Senator George C. Perkins in Washington, Governor Pardee estimated: "Three hundred million taxable property wiped out in San Francisco. . . ."[9] Others placed the loss at three times as high.

In the toll of major city monuments, the Chronicle and Call Buildings and the giant Emporium department store were lost. Of the storied mansions of Nob Hill tycoons—Stanford, Hopkins, Flood, Huntington, and Crocker—only scorched and hollow shells remained. Likewise, the Palace, the Fairmont, and the St. Francis also burned.

Tireless bucket brigades and employees beating embers with wet sacks saved the post office, courthouse, and U.S. Mint along Mission Street. Exhausted firefighters preserved the Ferry Building and the Southern Pacific Railroad Terminal, allowing over 200,000 refugees to flee by rail and sea.

The U.S. Army and city officials estimated that about 500 people had died. Later, historians calculated that the true toll of crushed and cremated humanity more closely approximated 3,000 lives.[10]

By the morning of Saturday, April 21, streams of seawater, favorable winds, and dynamited firebreaks finally starved the fire of fuel. In its wake, 490 blocks were incinerated. The homes of 250,000 San Franciscans were gone, along with libraries, courts, jails, theaters, restaurants, schools, churches, and centers of government and business. Communications and transportation systems were mute and paralyzed. And 10,000 of the city's gardens were a memory under ash and rubble.[11]

Over $8 million in relief monies were raised for relief of the place and its people. The actress Sarah Bernhardt gave benefit performances in Chicago and in Berkeley to help the city she loved. Donations ranged from bread to circuses: from loaves baked by students at an Indian school in Oregon to $200,000 in receipts from Barnum & Bailey. The undefeated boxing champion Jim Jeffries, cheered by thousands at the Mechanics' Pavilion, sold oranges for charity. Some service was compulsory: The actor John Barrymore was among those ordered to stack bricks by bayonet-wielding troops.[12]

Misery had a million faces. When George Houghton of Boston offered to donate a huge stock of footwear, it seemed a strange form of relief. But Governor Pardee eagerly accepted the gift. It turned out that many refugees had burned clean through their soles while walking across the hot cinders in city streets following the Great Fire.[13]

Hungry and begrimed, survivors huddled in a kind of democracy. Rich and poor dined from the same menu. The bill of fare included staple bread, canned meat, and potatoes distributed by 150 relief stations. The wealthy folks ate no better, for there was nothing to buy.

The volume of refugees numbered three hundred thousand on the night of April 18, when most of the city slept outdoors. By June, the population of refugee camps was down to fifty thousand. In the days to come, the census of refugees ebbed slowly as the city rebuilt itself. Still, there remained thousands in tents and dugouts, lean-tos and shacks, for many months.[14] The shelters barely kept out the elements. Blanket lean-tos were replaced by forests of military tents. Later, the city built thousands of two- and three-room wooden cottages. Occupants of the shelters cooked in communal kitchens and used earthen trenches or latrines for toilets. Flies bred and swarmed about the camps, and kitchens were hastily screened to prevent epidemics. Notices in English, Spanish, and Italian urged people to boil their water and milk.

In some people the temblor sparked a strange exhilaration. The philosopher William James, a visiting professor at Stanford University, was awed by its animal power. "Here at last was a *real* earthquake," he marveled, "after so many years of harmless waggle!" As the quake flung him about, he reflected, it shook the room "exactly as a terrier shakes a rat."[15]

Indeed, the earthquake shook thousands of rats from their hiding places. From fractured walls and ruptured sewer pipes, rats and fleas poured fourth, joining the river of refugees moving through the crumbled city. Like the human refugees, they too were fleeing the shattered remains of their homes.

Resourceful camp followers, the rats slowly made their way to the refugee camps. They flourished in the ruins, feasted off the garbage, and bred in abundance. The rodent diaspora set the stage for a new and unexpected aftershock of the earthquake.

As the telegraph machines in Washington chattered to life on the morning of April 18 with reports from San Francisco, Surgeon General Walter Wyman thought of Rupert Blue.

Blue was then in Washington to tackle a most unheroic temporary assignment: sanitary inspection of buildings in the nation's capital. It was an era when the halls of government had too many cockroaches and too few spittoons. But now there was a more urgent need for his services. While the Great Fire still smoldered, Blue boarded a train for the Pacific coast to assess the disaster.

On a ferry from Oakland, approaching the San Francisco waterfront, Blue scanned the shattered skyline for landmarks. As the shoreline came into focus, he could see the Ferry Building with its flagpole knocked askew and its clock hands frozen at just past five o'clock, the hour when the quake had hit. When the ferry docked, he emerged into streets that were buckled and filled with rubble. Mounds of bricks and masonry lay warped and blackened in the wake of the firestorm. Hills once terraced by houses and offices now bristled with jagged shells of scorched ruins. The dusty air smelled of pit latrines.

Prodigal and proud San Francisco now looked chastened, a town clad in sackcloth and ashes. The city he knew so well from its waterfront to its hilltops, Chinatown to the Latin Quarter, was a smoke-stained desert. Its features were scoured away, leaving a plain of blowing ash and sand. His father had witnessed cities leveled by the Civil War. What General Sherman did to the South, the earthquake did to San Francisco.

His first task was to visit refugee camps in the Mission district. With the streetcars stranded on their twisted rails, it was hard to find a buggy to navigate the debris-choked streets. On the slow, rocking ride, Blue saw Market Street with its grand hotels and shopping emporia hollowed out like a ghost town. South of the Market Street slot, he traversed a zone of smashed boardinghouses, slanted crazily on their foundations. But nothing prepared him for the spectacle of homeless masses camped out in the Mission district.

"Deplorable," he breathed under his mustache. "There must have been more than 30-thousand people living in shacks, tents, and other temporary abodes in this district. Those whose homes were spared have to cook in the streets, as all chimneys, water and sewer connections have been destroyed by the earthquake."[16] All through the city, the miserable scene was repeated ten times over.

Nothing stood between these refugees and disease outbreaks. Contaminated water, bad food, and overflowing latrines practically guaranteed an outbreak of "enteric," as Blue called typhoid fever.

In Dolores Park, refugees huddled in a hellish parody of summer camp. In a case of bad timing, city planners had planned a new lawn and spread the park soil with manure just before the earthquake hit. Now families with nowhere else to go built shanties and carved dugouts atop the malodorous mulch. There, they bedded down and cooked their rations.

And what rations. Cold mush and bad coffee were the morning bill of fare. Evenings, the lucky got stew and tea. The unlucky Larsen family in Fort Mason camp was issued a slab of flyblown meat, a bruised head of lettuce, withered radishes, and four potatoes stained with coal oil. Mrs. Larsen marched to the camp commander and complained that it was unfit for her brood of seven. The army officer in charge of city sanitation declined responsibility. Since the army didn't issue any fresh vegetables at all, he explained, the food couldn't have come from his operation.[17]

Refugees hoarded food in their tents, attracting hungry vermin. So the army ordered that all cooking be confined to communal kitchens.

But refugees set up the kitchens too close to the latrines, and many camps lacked screens to keep out the clouds of flies. The homeless on Telegraph Hill shunned the latrines and found relief in the shrubs, contaminating soil and groundwater. Garbage scavengers and latrine excavators were unreliable in their pickups and frequently dropped or scattered their collections. From the fractured sewer mains, rats scurried out to banquet on garbage heaps. They found sanctuary in the ruins, grew fat on the leftover rations, and bred furiously.

Soon camps were diagnosing refugees with cases of typhoid as well as scarlet fever, measles, mumps, diphtheria, and smallpox. Mass vaccination of the refugees began in the camps. Army doctors set up a smallpox hospital in Golden Gate Park, and tent clinics sprouted all over town.

Bedding, gauze, tents, food, and sanitary equipment rolled in by the ton. Along with all the standard disaster rations, the city's sanitary chief received this refreshing telegram from army headquarters in Washington: "Henry E. Netter, Philadelphia, has offered donation carload of eighty barrels rye whiskey for hospital purposes. Do you want it[?]" The medicinal spirits were shipped express.[18]

After checking the condition of the refugee camps, Blue had an unexpected encounter with his old nemesis. An Italian teenager in Oakland named Louis Scazzafava fell sick with a fever and aching, swollen glands. His sickness occurred just a few days after he'd gone hiking in the hills behind the Berkeley campus. Blue looked into the case. It was bubonic plague. However, it was a mild case, and with relief, Blue reported that the boy would live.

Blue's duties in the East were calling him back. He had the public health service's Norfolk station to look after. He also had the health and hygiene of the Jamestown Exposition under his command. President Roosevelt and the First Family were scheduled to preside over its grand opening, set for spring of 1907. It had to be perfect.

Still, he was reluctant to go. San Francisco's health seemed far from secure. The army and Red Cross were holding disaster at bay, although their pit latrines and diarrhea made life in the refugee camps an ordeal. Above all, he was troubled by his encounter with Louis Scazzafava, the teenage plague survivor. Plague wasn't his reason for coming west, but that was the memory that lingered.

"There seems nothing more for me to do here," Blue wrote to the surgeon general, "yet I am loth [*sic*] to leave in view of the possibility of plague among campers and pic-nic crowds in the Berkeley hills."[19]

Pushing aside his premonitions, Blue boarded a train back to his post in the East.

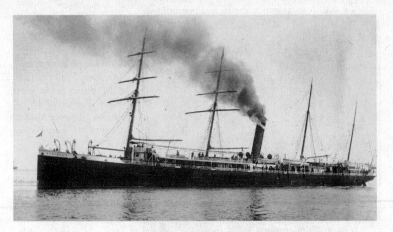

The *Australia*—the steamer that Quarantine Officer Joseph J. Kinyoun suspected brought plague into San Francisco. *John W. Procter Photographic Collection; courtesy of San Francisco Maritime National Historical Park*

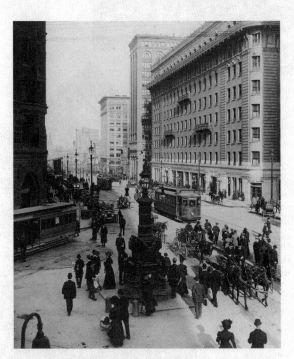

The intersection of Market and Kearny Streets in turn-of-the-century San Francisco. *Courtesy of the Society of California Pioneers*

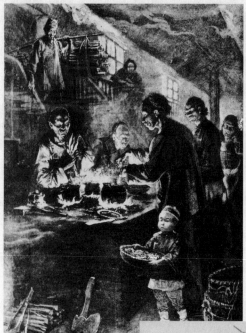

A drawing of a scene in Chinatown from the June 2, 1900, edition of *Harper's Weekly. Courtesy of the National Library of Medicine, History of Medicine Division*

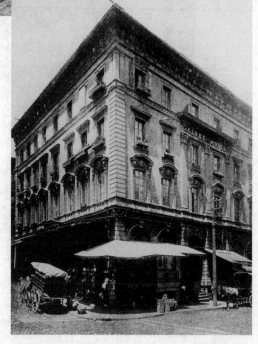

The Globe Hotel at Dupont and Jackson Streets in San Francisco's Chinatown, where Wong Chut King, the city's first plague victim, died in March 1900.
Courtesy of the San Francisco History Center, San Francisco Public Library

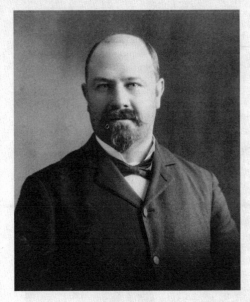

Bacteriologist Joseph Kinyoun (1860–1919), who served as quarantine officer in San Francisco and confirmed the presence of bubonic plague there. *Courtesy of the National Library of Medicine, History of Medicine Division*

Portrait of an older Kinyoun by Malmsley Lenhard. *Courtesy of the National Library of Medicine, History of Medicine Division*

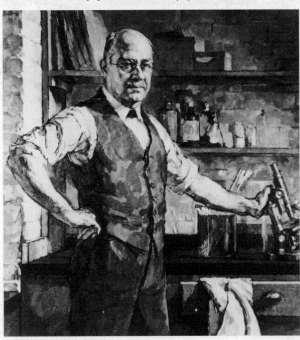

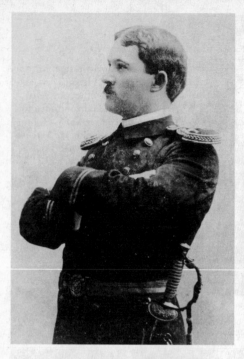

Dr. Rupert Lee Blue (1868–1948), in his twenties, in the uniform of the U.S. Marine Hospital Service. *Courtesy of South Caroliniana Library, University of South Carolina, Columbia*

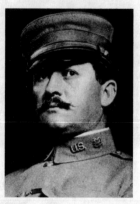

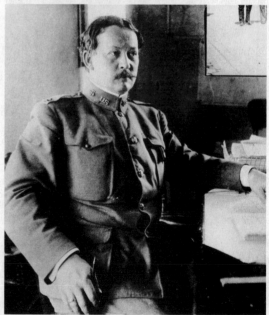

Blue at the time his plague campaign led him toward the post of surgeon general in 1912. *Courtesy of the San Francisco History Center, San Francisco Public Library*

Blue at his desk in San Francisco, circa 1909. *Courtesy of the National Library of Medicine, History of Medicine Division*

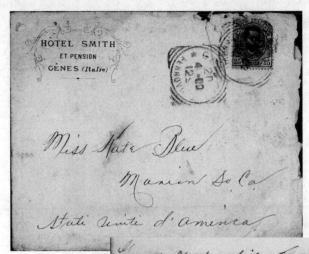

A letter from Rupert Blue to his sister Kate, sent from Italy, where he was posted by the U.S. Marine Hospital Service. *From the private collection of J. Michael Hughes*

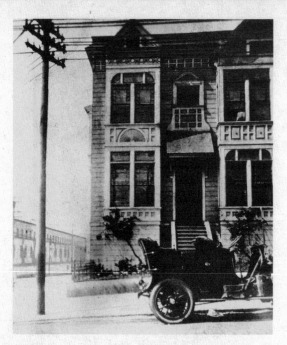

The Victorian house at 401 Fillmore Street that served as the plague campaign headquarters. *Courtesy of the National Library of Medicine, History of Medicine Division*

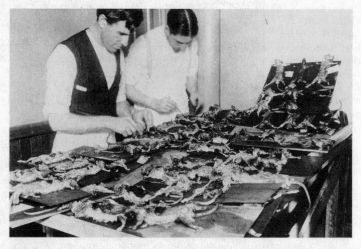

"The rattery," where rats were dissected, labeled, and nailed to shingles in an effort to detect bubonic plague. *Courtesy of the National Library of Medicine, History of Medicine Division*

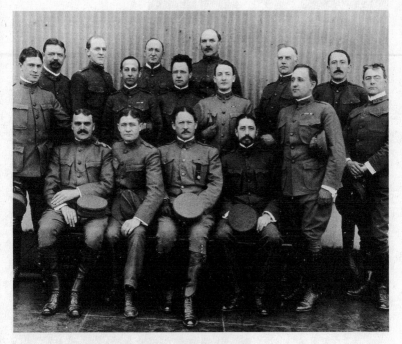

Rupert Blue (seated, second from right) with his officers, including Colby Rucker (standing, third from right) during the plague campaigns of 1907–1909.
Courtesy of the National Library of Medicine, History of Medicine Division

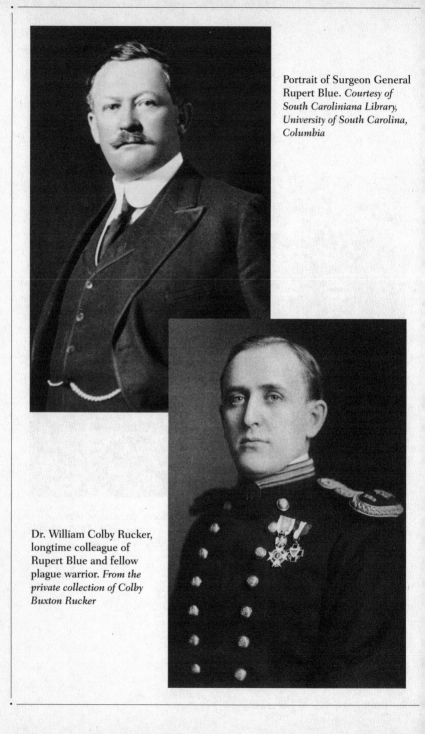

Portrait of Surgeon General Rupert Blue. *Courtesy of South Caroliniana Library, University of South Carolina, Columbia*

Dr. William Colby Rucker, longtime colleague of Rupert Blue and fellow plague warrior. *From the private collection of Colby Buxton Rucker*

"Comfort the People"

◉

IN 1907, SAN FRANCISCO ROSE phoenixlike from the rubble. The city was in such a rush to reinvent itself that it used firebricks, blistered survivors of the inferno, in construction. In Chinatown, these relics of the Great Fire stood out like dark scars on the fresh new facades.

Amid the upbeat clamor of construction, no one expected the trouble brewing aboard the tugboat *Wizard*. A seaman named Oscar Tomei had fallen ill. Stuporous with fever, Tomei was brought ashore and loaded into a buggy bound for the U.S. Marine Hospital. When he got there, Tomei lapsed into a coma. Burning and mute, he couldn't give doctors any clue to how he'd caught the infection swimming in his blood.

Bacillus pestis, the plague bacteria. On May 29, Tomei died.

Disbelief, then fear, gripped the doctors. Wasn't plague wiped out three years ago? They scrambled to interview Tomei's shipmates about his illness, but the *Wizard* and its crew were gone. The tug had steamed out the Golden Gate and headed north up the Mendocino coast. Word came that the *Wizard* sank in high seas, taking Tomei's history to the bottom of the ocean.

Plague was back in San Francisco, its origins unknown. Now a new team presided over the crisis: Governor George Pardee was ousted after his supporters in the Southern Pacific Railroad Co. cooled toward his independent style. The railroad switched its support to a rural congressman, James N. Gillett, who was elected governor with the help of that old San Francisco kingmaker Boss Abe Ruef.[1]

Ruef's own political star was sputtering out, too. Muckraking newspapermen and graft-weary politicians teamed up to evict the corrupt administration from City Hall. They asked President Roosevelt's help in enlisting a famous Secret Service agent, William Burns, and a special prosecutor, Francis Heney, to probe the payoffs. Ruef maintained his innocence until he was indicted on sixty-five counts of bribery. Then he pleaded guilty and testified against his old protégé Mayor Schmitz—ensuring felony convictions for both.[2]

With Ruef and Schmitz headed for jail, the city appointed as mayor a respected attorney and physician, Edward R. Taylor, who they hoped could heal City Hall from the inside out.

For ten weeks after Oscar Tomei's death, plague went silent. Then on August 12, the peace was shattered by a telephone call to the city board of health. Physician Guido Caglieri called from his office at Broadway and Kearny to report a desperately sick young Italian couple in his care.

Francesco Conti and his wife, Ida, were laid up with high fevers and crushing headaches in their house at 20 Midway in the Latin Quarter. The doctor administered fever remedies, which in that day ran the gamut from aspirin to arsenic, from lemonade to opium. Their fevers fell and then rose again to 104 degrees. Only then did the doctor discover the mirror-image lumps that protruded from Francesco's right groin and Ida's left thigh. He called an ambulance. The Conti house was quarantined, their child placed with charity child services.

Francesco, clinging to life, was carried to the City and County Hospital isolation ward. He would live. For his wife, it was too late. The infection overflowed from her bursting lymph glands, poisoning her bloodstream in an overwhelming sepsis. Under the germ's assault, her blood pressure fell, and in this state of shock, her organs failed. By the time the ambulance arrived, Ida was dead.

At that moment, across town, the doctors at the Marine Hospital were hovering over another dying sailor. This time it was a crew member from the steamer *Samoa*. Just twenty-one years old, Alexander Ruvak wheezed like an ancient marine. His agonal gasps left a ruby froth on his lips. When his struggle ended in death, the doctors were ready to list simple pneumonia on his death certificate. Then they noticed the lumps on his neck—suspicious symptoms that called for an autopsy. From both his lungs and his glands, the doctors extracted fluid swimming with plague bacteria.

The next day was August 13. At the clapboard City and County Hospital, doctors hovered over two newly admitted patients. Guadalupe Mendoza and Jose Hyman, Spanish laborers in their twenties, had been housemates, sharing a Pacific Street shack on the waterfront, where rats congregated. When the fever struck them down, the men were brought to the hospital, where no amount of care could save them.

As their bodies were prepared for autopsy, a sixty-three-year-old Irish-born orderly named Jeremiah O'Leary was on duty on the ward. His hand had an open wound.

By the time the doctors finished their autopsy and figured out what had killed Mendoza and Hyman, the orderly O'Leary had a rising temperature.

A tremor of terror passed through the isolation wards as word spread that the orderly had contracted plague from a patient. A nervous young intern named Arthur Reinstein panicked and refused to tend to O'Leary.

Pale and agitated, Reinstein submitted a letter of resignation, citing "obvious reasons." The city health board fired him for moral cowardice and neglect of duty. The orderly O'Leary died after a swift two-day siege. Reinstein later begged to return to work, got reinstated, and then resigned again—this time for good.[3]

Rats infiltrated the wards of the City and County Hospital, but their presence wasn't noticed until a patient, who came to the hospital to get well, got sicker instead. A forty-year-old Irish-born laborer named John Casey was admitted for a routine illness. While in his hospital bed, he contracted bubonic plague from the unseen vermin. Next, a nurse and intern at the hospital contracted plague.

The hospital was now hopelessly contaminated. Quarantined on August 27, it closed its doors to all but plague patients. The majority of the sick were loaded onto ambulances and transferred to the city almshouse overlooking a tiny lake, Laguna Honda. In a desperate attempt to keep the rats out and the plague in, the hospital tried to erect an iron fence around its infectious diseases pavilion, but local laborers, frightened that they would be the next victims, refused to work. Doctors were forced to do double duty as construction workers.[4]

The city carted in tons of sulfur and ignited five hundred smudge pots. The rank and choking clouds helped but couldn't purge the infestation. A horrified health board member reported, "The rats have so many runways through the hospital and have burrowed so deep even under the soil; into the sills of the building. The sewers are filled and the foundation is full of them. Sulphur [*sic*] does not penetrate sufficiently to destroy all the rats."[5]

Unlike his predecessors, Mayor Edward Taylor wasted no time in alerting the president and asking for help. He telegraphed Theodore Roosevelt, requesting that the Public Health and Marine Hospital Service send officers to the city's aid, pledging his cooperation and city funds to help them stop the outbreak.

President Roosevelt was savoring the end of summer at his estate on Oyster Bay, Long Island, when he got the telegram. On September 5, he wired Surgeon General Walter Wyman, ordering him to take action at once.[6]

The surgeon general telegraphed Mayor Taylor that he was putting his most experienced man in charge. "Passed Assistant Surgeon Blue," he said, "will leave Washington tomorrow for San Francisco."[7]

As Blue prepared to leave Virginia for San Francisco, Colby Rucker, the ablest of his junior officers and one of his closest friends, begged Blue to take him to San Francisco to join in the epidemic campaign. In a few days, Rucker received his orders, too, and set out for the Golden Gate with Annette and their young son.[8]

The public health service already had several men on the ground in San Francisco, preparing for their arrival. Among them was thirty-two-year-old bacteriologist Halstead Stansfield. Stansfield was a widower who had buried his wife and baby daughter the year before. Uncontrolled grief had deepened into melancholy, and he often drank himself numb. But still he roused himself to canvas the city for a plague laboratory and make it ready for the campaign.

As Blue's train clattered across the continent, past the Mississippi River, the Rockies, the Great Salt Lake, and the Sierras, the plague toll grew at a steady pace. Each day of his journey, it claimed a different life in a different part of town: from a hotel clerk on Hyde Street to an unemployed man on Harrison in the area south of Market Street.

Plague was a different beast in 1907 from what it was in 1900. This time its attack was different. In 1900, it had focused on one small neighborhood. Now there were widespread multiple outbreaks, with cases cropping up all over town, from the waterfront in the northeast to the County Hospital in the southwest. In 1900, the plague seemed to target the Chinese. In 1907, it attacked San Franciscans of many races. Still, old myths died hard, said a local historian, Frank Morton Todd. "It was curious how hard these ideas were to dispel, even in the face of the evidence furnished by white men's funerals."[9]

The disease's old target, Chinatown, seemed to be spared the onslaught—with one notable exception: the sixty-three-year-old president of the Chinese Six Companies. Chin Mon Way, a native of China, died suddenly, leaving his wife a widow and his trade organization leaderless. Word of his death touched off panic among the people who remembered the outbreak in 1900. They consulted the Chinese newspapers to ask if the epidemic had returned to their corner of the city. The Chinatown daily, *Chung Sai Yat Po*, reported Chin's death but treated the plague diagnosis with skepticism. The deaths this time are concentrated among the Caucasians, the paper said. The Chinese were urged to remain calm.[10]

The following day, on September 12, Blue arrived in San Francisco just as plague took another life, that of a twenty-two-year-old Greek laborer on Green Street. By the time he reported for duty, the toll stood at twenty-five cases, thirteen deaths.

Blue saw a San Francisco still crippled but gamely limping back to life. Freshly sawn timber frames stood over the razed ruins. Stores hung impromptu banners over temporary headquarters. He felt the resolute buoyancy of the citizenry. But he also saw a city ripe for epidemic: Forty thousand earthquake refugees camped in sordid shacks, two-thirds of the city lacked sewerage, and many streets lay buckled and impassable.

In Union Square, charred shells of hotels ringed the bronze *Victory* statue, who still held her wreath and trident aloft as she had when Roosevelt dedicated her in 1903. Under her lithe figure, more nymph than battle goddess, Blue put down his suitcase at "the Little

St. Francis," a makeshift wooden hostelry with space for one hundred guests. The main Hotel St. Francis, despite its "fireproof" label, had been completely gutted by flames.[11]

Stansfield greeted Blue with bad news. Nobody wanted to rent space for the public health service headquarters and plague laboratory. Landlords were squeamish about a band of scientists sharing their tenancy with the germs of a deadly epidemic. Downtown remained shattered. The business center had migrated west of Van Ness to Fillmore Street. Office space—where it existed at all—was scarce. Moreover, the traveling lab gear that had been shipped express to San Francisco had been lost in transit.

Blue met the city health board at its temporary headquarters on O'Farrell and Scott Streets. He listened in silence as the board fretted that the mayor's call for help would trigger a renewed quarantine. Bled by reconstruction costs, the city couldn't afford another fiscal blow. Blue helped them draft a message to inform and to calm the citizens:

> *To the People of San Francisco:*
> *Rumors of an alarming nature having reached the board of health in regard to bubonic plague, the president of the board, by its authority, hereby declares that there exists at present in San Francisco nothing that need cause any alarm, much less the quarantining of the city, and that there is at present no intention to make such quarantine.*
>
> *So far there have been detected but 25 verified cases of the disease since the 27th day of May last. Every precaution is being taken by the federal authorities, in co-operation with the state and city boards of health to stamp out such of the disease as is here. It is well to bear in mind that the bubonic plague seldom becomes epidemic except in the tropics.*[12]

The statement's plague count was true. But its breezy tone concealed wishful thinking. Rupert Blue's report to Surgeon General Wyman paints a picture at odds with his calming words to the citizens.

"Rats abound in large numbers in the whole city, particularly in the burned district, where conditions for their maintenance are ideal.

The ruins and piles of building material, and the broken and choked sewers form excellent nesting places, while the warehouses and uncollected garbage furnish an unlimited food supply. In addition, the houses for the most part are unprotected against the ingress of rats and other vermin," he wrote.

"The section in which the foci are most numerous contain the refugee camps which are built up in many places of shacks, and flea-infested cottages. The camps which are under the direction of the Relief Committee are in good sanitary condition, but they are in close proximity to the warehouses and broken sewers, which harbor large numbers of rats. . . . There are still many pit latrines in use. . . . The city is very dusty. . . .

"The widespread area of the disease indicates that the campaign will be a long and expensive one, and the available City fund will be rapidly expended."[13]

THE BOARD OF SUPERVISORS DUG deep and appropriated $25,000 from the dwindling city treasury to pay the plague expenses for September and pledged $20,000 a month after that. Blue said the public health service would place twelve medical men, and the city agreed to employ thirty-six sanitary inspectors. This was the seed of the corps.

After canvassing the city, the federal plague laboratory finally found a home in a two-story Victorian house at 401 Fillmore near Haight Street, rented from Mrs. M. M. Fitzgerald for $80 a month. Set on a ridge of middle-class frame houses, the plague laboratory hung out a sign and began hiring a motley crew of rat catchers and sanitary engineers. Jobless men flocked to apply. Under a plan devised by Japanese plague pioneer Kitasato, the city was divided into twelve plague districts, each under the direction of a public health service doctor to oversee the raw recruits.

The city, despite its poverty, managed a gallant gesture. To make it easier for Blue to navigate the fractured streets of the city on his daily rounds, the city offered him a motorcar for his official use. So he now had access to those places the streetcars couldn't go.

The old City and County Hospital was condemned. The isolation ward for plague patients was being moved from the original site to a new rat-proof compound ringed by eight feet of galvanized steel at Army and De Haro Streets. The exodus of other patients had already taken them to far-flung sites around town: the Presidio Hospital, the almshouse, private hospitals. Even the horse stalls at Ingleside Racetrack—abandoned as too drafty for Thoroughbreds—sheltered the sick and aged.[14]

Conditions citywide were ideal for an explosion of plague. The lone bright spot, Blue boasted, was Chinatown, where plague was almost nonexistent. He attributed this to his campaign back in 1903 and 1904 to build out the plague with cement basements in the district.

For some reason, Chinatown's mistrust now began to soften. Unlike the "wolf doctor," Joseph Kinyoun, the soft-spoken Blue won over the community by degrees. The *Chung Sai Yat Po,* the Greek chorus of the neighborhood, signaled its approval of the new commander:

Dr. Blue, who was sent by Washington to investigate the plague, said it is not serious. People should not be frightened, he said. They will not overdo the quarantining of the houses, or harass the residents. Their main emphasis is to go after the rats. These physicians are very kind and gentle. They told our reporter to comfort the people.[15]

The Rattery

◉

BLUE HAD NO ILLUSIONS. "The campaign is likely to be a long one," he warned a colleague in Washington, "and the infestation will be fifty times more difficult of eradication than before. The foci are to be found all over the city, the greater number existing in the burned district where, on account of the protection afforded by the ruins, the rats multiply in countless numbers. . . . The people are very much alarmed [and] fear a quarantine. . . ."[1]

At 401 Fillmore Street, Blue organized his command center and the federal laboratory. Tucked into a nondescript annex behind the Victorian headquarters stood the heart of the operation—"the rattery." The rattery held narrow lead-topped dissection tables, covered in rodent carcasses that were split tip to tail for postmortem analysis. Tacked on the walls of the rattery were sticky rectangles of flypaper to trap any insects that might alight on a rat and then buzz away to spread the germs. It was like a coroner's office for rats.

Aproned men in shirtsleeves—sometimes gloved—skinned and dipped each carcass in disinfectant. Each rat was numbered, nailed on a shingle, and labeled with the date and address of its capture. With quick, light blade strokes, the men made a long vertical incision, gently, to avoid damaging internal organs. Peering into the split thorax and abdomen, they searched for signs that mirrored human plague symptoms: swollen glands about the throat, enlarged hearts, livers, or spleens. Any sign of infection triggered a further round of tests.

The men summoned Stansfield when they found signs of plague. He then snipped minuscule tissue samples of glands, spleen, or liver. From these, he prepared glass slides for the microscope. He also dotted samples onto culture plates containing a nutrient broth resembling an overripe dish of jellied consommé. Then he watched the culture dish to see if the samples would sprout germ colonies with a ground-glass texture, spreading and thickening into plaques with a pattern that resembled beaten copper—the look of plague bacteria colonies. He injected the germs into guinea pigs and waited to see if the animals lived or died. On such tests, the city's future health depended.

It was a bloody, reeking business. The rat crews were skinning, splitting, and examining rats as fast as they could. As their speed and efficiency grew, the crews dissected hundreds of rats a day. Each day they filled eight to ten steel garbage cans with split carcasses, which were carted off to be burned in the incinerator. The rank and musky scent clung to their clothes and nostrils. It took bars of strong soap, dousings with eau de cologne, and snifters of brandy to rid themselves of the reek of it at day's end.

It was always a dangerous operation. Although any rats caught live could be plunged into boiling water, drowned in kerosene, or gassed with formaldehyde, there was always a chance that some stray flea might leap off its doomed host in time to bite the unwary inspector. And for this reason, the men took injections of vaccine or antiserum.

With the growing harvest, Blue's men acquired an intimate knowledge of the domestic life of *Rattus norvegicus*. The Norway rat—also known as the brown rat or sewer rat—is a bulky hunch-backed brute with a small head and naked scaly tail. A prolific breeder, it beats its smaller seagoing cousin *Rattus rattus* (aka the shipboard rat or roof rat) in fecundity. Blue and Rucker analyzed the enemy:

We have found in our work that a rat-run usually branches like a Y. At one extremity of the fork is a little store-house in which may be found corn, wheat, pieces of bread and apple cores. At the other end is the nest made of rags and feathers laid on straw or hay and offering an ideal breeding place for fleas. This display of ingenuity and foresight gives us a clew [*sic*] to another characteristic of the rat, namely his sagacity . . .

when man begins to fight the rat it is a battle between the intelligence of the one and the instinct of the other with the advantage not always on the side of the former.[2]

Every day, the laborers hit the streets, searching houses, placing poisons, closing rat holes, and burning garbage. Medical inspectors made rounds to inspect the sick and the dead. Most plague patients were taken to the county's plague camp—a few blocks from the old condemned hospital—or to its morgue.

The link between rats, people, and plague now captured more of Rupert Blue's attention. Even during the first outbreak, he'd operated on the assumption that controlling vermin was a key to controlling plague. Only now did the precise role of fleas start to emerge from the shadows.

Blue wrote Washington asking them to send him literature on the spread of plague in India and China. In 1906 the doctors of the plague commission in India and others had just begun to publish their confirmations of what French researcher Paul-Louis Simond had discovered a decade earlier—that a flea bite could spread plague germs. Surgeon General Wyman, recognizing this as a landmark observation, had begun circulating the reports to his men up and down the West Coast in early 1907.

Poring over those reports, Blue began to refine his attack. Rats were the agents of epidemic, dealing death by means of the insects that hid in their pelts. Now Blue began to push his men to autopsy more and more rats every day, as many as the rattery could handle. He began to understand and anticipate the alternating seasons of rat plague and human plague, mediated by a tiny go-between: a glossy brown bloodsucker no bigger than a sesame seed.

The peak season for human plague ran from April to September, Blue observed, coinciding with the balmy months when fleas flourished, bred, and fed avidly. Then from October to March, cold would descend, and the fleas would hibernate. But these winter doldrums were deceiving, for it was high season for rat plague. Wet weather makes them loath to leave their burrows for food, and they turn to cannibalism. Sick members of the colony are defenseless against their predatory kin. As they feed on one another, the infection spreads. In spring, warmth lures the rats into the open just when flea eggs hatch.

The cycle begins anew and lasts through the warmth of a San Francisco autumn, until the chilly bands of rain sweep in off the Pacific, driving vermin underground.

After less than a month on site, Blue's October 3 tally of human plague showed fifty-one positive cases, forty-four suspicious cases, and thirty deaths. With the rats flourishing and the sickness increasing, Blue needed to enlist the city in his campaign. He drafted a circular to be delivered to every home, business, warehouse, factory, bakery, restaurant, and hotel in town. Set out traps and poison, he urged. Plug up rat holes. Seal garbage in metal cans. Make every building rat-proof. He avoided the word *plague*. The Merchants' Association liked this soft sell and sent Blue's circular to every address in San Francisco.[3]

Of all the stricken blocks in San Francisco, none was more infected than Lobos Square. A refugee camp in the Marina district, Lobos Square was a gridlike village of 750 wooden earthquake cottages built by the Red Cross to shelter two thousand homeless people. It was so vast that it had its own numbered streets and addresses. It also attracted its own resident rats.

The rats slipped into the wooden cottages, their pelts alive with fleas. The fleas alighted on sixteen-month-old Mary Costello, puncturing her tender skin. The toddler fussed and scratched the bite, working the germs deeper into the bite wound. Days later, fever and ominous swellings arose. She died on September 27. A neighbor child, five-year-old Thomasa Herrera, died two weeks later. Living as refugees, dying of epidemic, the girls had few to mourn them. According to city death certificates, their parents were unknown. They were among the camp's eighteen plague victims.

The next week, on October 18, Blue sent an update in code: "*Bumpkin to date: positive sixty five, suspicious thirty eight, deaths thirty eight. . . .*"[4] Sixty-five cases of confirmed plague, thirty-eight suspicious cases, and thirty-eight dead. Blue usually sent encrypted dispatches under his own name instead of his heroic-sounding code name, "*Achieving.*"

The rat eradication program was costing $30,000 to $50,000 a month for salaries for his dozen medical officers, wages for three hundred laborers, thousands of traps, tons of cheese bait and mountains of poison, plus the rent on the Victorian headquarters. But the city could ill afford to help; every coin in the municipal coffers was earmarked to mend the earthquake-ruined streets and sewers. Blue haggled with Washington for funds. After his long-lost lab set arrived, smashed in transit, Blue was denied the $250 to replace it. He was ordered to get competitive bids. Federal protocols ground slowly.

Back in Washington from a trip abroad, Surgeon General Walter Wyman leafed through the reports from San Francisco. He was furious—not about the plague, but about Blue's bookkeeping. He dashed off a stinging critique, demanding that reports be sent in a carefully prescribed style and format.

Blue absorbed this rebuke. It was clear the surgeon general had no notion of the disaster Blue was just barely holding at bay: a city shattered, crawling with rats, deeply plague infested, tended by an unreliable labor force of strikers and political hacks. Blue tidied his reports, swore to unify his men, and drove them to boost their catch—first 1,000 rats a day, then 1,200 rats a day.[5]

As the rattery's operations grew, and as Mayor Edward Taylor readied a delegation to plead for federal aid, Secretary of the Treasury George B. Cortelyou relented. The federal government agreed to bear plague expenses of $50,000 a month. Washington's promised cash infusion came none too soon. The contagion of fear was spreading overseas. In late October, the kingdom of Norway declared a quarantine against San Francisco, Secretary of State Elihu Root told the cabinet. On October 29, Blue reported that San Francisco had counted seventy-eight positive cases of plague, thirty-five suspicious cases, and fifty deaths.

Blue escalated his war on rats. On November 8, he wrote to Surgeon General Wyman that his weekly catch reached a new high of thirteen thousand rats. Still more rats lay dead of plague or poison, hidden in labyrinths under city streets. The sewer men had never seen so many.

But thanks to the rats' legendary procreative power, they were now breeding faster than they could be trapped. A female rat bears ten to fifteen pups every four months. The pups mature quickly and begin to breed at the age of four months. By the end of a year, one family can produce eight hundred rats. The quake ruins served as both honeymoon bower and nursery. The explosion in the rat population was echoed by a flea baby boom. In winter, Blue observed, his men could comb twenty rats and find only one flea among them. But in warm weather, everything changed: One healthy rat could harbor twenty-five fleas, while a sick one could carry eighty-five.

Amid all these multiplying vermin, everyone in town, rich and poor, was put in harm's way. Not even the medical profession was immune. The family of a physician identified in records only as "Dr. C." noticed a high, sweet, sickening odor wafting from the walls of their second-story flat. To root out the source of the stench, the doctor tore out the wainscoting around some plumbing lines. There inside a hollow wall lay two rats in an advanced state of putrefaction. Removing them from the wall took care of the smell, but it was a risky operation. Days later, one family member was dead of plague, and another was critically ill. After an investigation, Blue concluded that rat fleas, which had been trapped and starving on the dead rats in the wall, took advantage of the doctor's remodeling to escape and prey on his family for their next warm-blooded meal.[6]

Playing with rats was even deadlier for a family in the Mission district. One day in November, two young Bowers brothers were playing in an unused cellar when they made a thrilling find: a furry rat corpse. After entombing the rat in a shoebox coffin, the brothers performed a funeral service and buried the animal. The macabre game was natural enough, given the profession of their father: Otis Howard Bowers was an undertaker.

Following their solemn service, the boys raced home for dinner at 2888 Mission Street, a strip of Victorian flats over shops along the clamorous commercial thoroughfare named for the white Spanish adobe church of Mission Dolores nearby.

The boys unwittingly brought home a souvenir of their secret game: fleas. The parasites leapt unseen from the rat cadaver onto the children's legs and hitchhiked home, where the boys rejoined their parents, their grandmother, and their little sister.

Insidiously, the infection took hold. The first to feel its effects was the thirty-seven-year-old father of the family, who discovered a tender lump on his right thigh. Soon, a fever and crushing fatigue forced him to bed. As his wife and mother-in-law hovered around the sickroom, Mr. Bowers grew insensible of his surroundings.

With her husband febrile and unresponsive, a frightened Margaret Bowers called for a doctor. By this time, her husband's illness was so advanced that the doctor could offer little to help. The infection overflowed from his lymph glands into his bloodstream, throwing him into irreversible shock and organ failure. An hour after the doctor's visit, Bowers was dead.

By now, one of his boys, three-year-old Joseph, had sprouted a painful lump in his left thigh. The little boy was put in a carriage and taken to the isolation hospital.

Two nights after Howard Bowers died, his widow plunged into a profound malaise. Neighbors might have mistaken her misery for deep mourning. But it wasn't grief alone that blanched her cheeks and reddened her eyes. Pain pounded her skull and raked her back and limbs. Despite the cool of late fall, fever cloaked her corset in clammy sweat.

When doctors arrived the next morning, they found Margaret Bowers very weak. Her bloodshot gaze was baleful, and her face was a mask of pain and fear—the "pestlike expression" that doctors now saw as a sign of plague. During examination, doctors discovered a mass of swollen, tender glands in her left thigh. Doctors gathered up her limp form, bundled her into a horse-drawn ambulance, and carted her to the isolation hospital, where her three-year-old Joseph lay fighting for his life. There she was admitted and injected with massive amounts of Yersin's antiserum, her only hope of withstanding the infection. In a nearby bed, the resilient Joseph began to improve.

Meanwhile, at home, Mrs. Bowers's two-year-old daughter and her sixty-year-old mother, Bridget Noiset, developed ominous fevers and swellings. The toddler and her grandmother were now admitted to the hospital with a diagnosis of bubonic plague. A third Bowers child was hospitalized, but he alone managed to evade the voracious fleas and stay healthy.

Confined in a county hospital isolation cottage, Mrs. Bowers seemed to respond to the antiserum infusions. Her fever wavered and dipped. Doctors hoped she could outlast the siege. But she still complained of an ache beneath her left breast and ribs.

Sudddenly, on the evening of December 6, Margaret Bowers's fever shot up to 104 degrees. The germs had flowed through her bloodstream, colonizing her lungs. Now she had pneumonic plague.

As she fought to breathe, the bacteria and debris from dead cells clogged the air sacs of her lungs. Her blood frothed but failed to pick up any oxygen. Each breath was labored; she starved for air. On December 8, with her little boy recuperating nearby and her helpless nurses looking on, Margaret Bowers suffocated. Her heart stopped in midcontraction. She was twenty-seven years old.[7]

The Bowers boys, now orphaned, told the doctors of their dead rat discovery, its mock funeral, and the cardboard tomb. Investigators backtracked to Mission Street, unearthed the coffin, and transported the rat to the plague laboratory at 401 Fillmore Street. There, Blue's team split, skinned, and autopsied the animal. No one was surprised to find the bacteria of plague.[8] An innocent game had killed the boys' parents.

Not until the second plague was under way did San Francisco address the rats' portal of entry: the waterfront. Although ships had long been fumigated, few barriers had prevented the rats from scuttling between ship and shore. Now at Blue's urging, the city began to order the building of metal and concrete wharves and piers, replacing the old, rat-ridden wood pilings. On the hawsers that moored ships to the docks, shippers placed new effective rat guards, some with traps, to thwart the four-legged stowaways. Meanwhile, on dry land, Blue and Rucker refined their training of the rat-catcher corps.

"A man can no more be made into a rat-catcher by giving him a rat trap than he can become a soldier by being provided with a rifle," Blue wrote.[9] He was concerned that his own crew was being undermined by the shoddy and dispirited local laborers they'd hired to catch rats. Many of the men were out-of-work streetcar operators and political hangers-on who had signed up thinking they wouldn't have to break a sweat. So Blue imposed a merit system, firing the slackers and rewarding the diligent with pay raises. He also transformed rat catching into a precise science.

His executive officer, W. Colby Rucker, wrote a detailed treatise titled "How to Catch Rats." Take a nineteen-inch French wire trap, placed where rats come to drink, and camouflage it with a layer of hay, straw, or wood, he advised. Then tempt the beasts with an ever-changing smorgasbord of raw meat, cheddar cheese, smoked fish, fresh liver, corned beef, fried bacon, pine nuts, apples, carrots, and corn. Scatter a trail of barley to attract animals to the trap. Smoke the trap with a burning newspaper to mask the telltale scent of human hands. As an added lure, place a small chick or duckling nearby to peep enticingly. When a female rat is caught, leave her in the trap so her cries will summon her suitors and offspring. However, Rucker warned, "It is not wise to kill rats where they are caught, as the squealing may frighten the other rats away."[10] So irresistible was Rucker's regimen that hundreds of thousands of rats were drawn to their doom.

Khaki-uniformed public health officers patrolled the city's thirteen plague districts—Blue had added one more district as if to mock superstition, Colby said. The men were becoming a familiar sight to the San Francisco citizenry. Public antagonism now softened a bit. Perhaps overconfidently, Blue chose this moment to venture into the heart of his opposition.

Making an appointment at the editorial offices of the *San Francisco Chronicle,* Blue requested an audience with Michael Harry de Young. M. H. de Young—an autocratic publisher, Republican power broker, and disappointed Senate hopeful—long had linked the city's fortunes with his own. A passionate and prodigious collector, he gave the city its first public art gallery, the De Young Museum in Golden Gate Park. As a lover of beautiful things, the fifty-eight-year-old publisher found no place in his city for anything as hideous as an epidemic. After surviving an attempted assassination and an earthquake, he wouldn't countenance quarantine. Nor was he about to have his paper's editorial policy dictated by a federal bureaucrat who would destroy the city for the sake of a scientific theory.

"We need your help," Blue beseeched. He begged the publisher to offer his readers factual reports on the plague. Without that, the public health service could not engage the support of the people in the gritty business of rat eradication. De Young's face was opaque, his reply cold and noncommittal. He was used to being courted *before* a program was launched. Blue's mission was a failure.

"I had an interview with Mr. De Young," wrote the crestfallen plague commander to Washington. "He is a strange, stubborn man and may turn his guns on us with greater effect than ever." However, he noted, "The city authorities, press and people, with the single exception of the *Chronicle,* seem to be with us heart and soul."[11]

Back at the rattery on Fillmore Street, Stansfield and other officers were drained. Yet only a fraction of the lab tests Blue needed was getting done. Fewer than two hundred rats a day were being examined for the infection. He needed more data. The nests of plague—both human and rodent—were so widespread that only three of the city's thirteen districts remained free from infection.

Just after Thanksgiving, the plague toll reached 106 confirmed cases and 65 deaths. Outwardly, Blue kept up his can-do outlook. His men needed him to be a perfect model of the "sanitarian spirit." But in private, Blue was anything but cocky.

Blue was late sending funds to his mother and sisters in South Carolina. A bank panic triggered by Washington's trust-busting made it difficult to buy a draft. So he wrote promising to send his next paycheck home in its entirety and gave his family a report on his progress. "My campaign is showing marked results in reducing the number of cases," he wrote Annie Maria. But he added, "We have yet a great work to do this winter."[12]

Seven days a week, the lights in the mullioned windows of 401 Fillmore Street burned into the night. Weekends and holidays did not interrupt Blue's calendar. He drove his men hard. They thought him insatiable, a zealot. But remarkably, few men had complained so far. Hundreds of laborers laid thousands of traps, baited with tons of cheese, every month. But the rats still flourished, and the deaths still rose.

By the end of 1907, doctors had diagnosed 136 people with plague and buried 73 of them—almost all in four months. That December, Blue sent Washington a grim prediction for the New Year:

"Conditions are not improving as rapidly as I would like them to. . . . There can be no doubt that the city is infected from one end to the other," he said. He felt his campaign was at a crossroads: Rid the city of rats by winter's end or face "an outbreak of unprecedented proportions."[13]

But despite the months of strenuous rat work, eradication seemed as far off as ever. In the war room of his headquarters on Fillmore Street, Rupert Blue paged through medical journals for clues to the plague's next move. In Manila, when just 2 percent of rats became infected, it ignited an explosive epidemic among the populace. Among San Francisco's rats, his tests showed that the infection rate was 1.5 percent and rising.

His mission was to exterminate all the rats before the infection rate in San Francisco reached this trigger point. He seized worksheets for the week ended January 11, 1908, and ticked off the figures:

352,000 bits of poisoned bait placed, and thousands of rats collected from traps and the bounty program. He was disheartened to see that the rats' infection rate had tripled since the fall.

They would have to work harder. Spring was coming on fast. They had little time before new litters of baby rats and hungry hatchling fleas would emerge, ensuring that plague would bloom again.

The logjam in the lab was intolerable, Blue decided. It was moving too slowly; they were testing just one-third of the burgeoning daily rat catch. It was simple: Stansfield must speed up.

Pushing past the glass doors, Blue entered the lab in search of his bacteriologist. There amid the vials and flasks, bathed in the yeasty smell of his bacteria broth, sat Halstead Stansfield. Blue found it hard to choke back his impatience. The lab was falling behind; it needed to run more tests. "I need a trained assistant," Stansfield replied wearily. Blue replied he'd already asked the surgeon general; the request had been vetoed on budgetary grounds.

Instead of soldiering on, Stansfield was giving up and giving in to his demons. Chronically melancholy, soured by hangover, he'd erupt in a rage when his fellow officers tried to buck him up. Stansfield was still grieving over the deaths of his wife and child. Blue was sorry for his loss, but he had an epidemic to fight.

As if work weren't troubled enough, an unforeseen accident almost derailed the rat eradication campaign. It was bound to happen in a town as studded with rat bait as a panettone is with raisins. Three children at play spied what looked like a picnic in a French wire basket. Morsels of bread and cheese were buttered with a puree they did not recognize. The children bit into the purloined snack and instantly regretted it.

It was laced with Stearns' Electric Rat and Roach Paste, containing phosphorous poison, which burns the mucous membranes and leaves a searing trail down one's throat and stomach. Though wretchedly sick, the children survived. Had they died, the campaign might have died with them.

Blue ordered a ban on phosphorous poison. It was simply too dangerous to use in a densely populated city. The campaign would switch to Danysz virus, the germ that was fatal to rodents but harmless to people. Blue instructed the laboratory at 401 Fillmore to brew up extra-strength batches of the stuff at once.

Once again, Stansfield balked. He now spent days at a time away from his lodgings at the Majestic Hotel. Drowning his grief in alcohol, he was deaf to the pleas of his fellow officers. The lab work languished. Blue had no choice but to ask that Washington replace Stansfield. "I have no hope of a change in him. I have exhausted patience in reasoning with him," Blue wrote to Assistant Surgeon General Glennan. "The work and the campaign have become so exacting that I scarcely have time to eat and sleep properly, I simply cannot have a controversy with an officer at this time."[14]

But Colby Rucker was performing admirably as Blue's right-hand man. Installed in a modest residential hotel with his wife, Annette, and young son, Colby, he played dominoes and entertained his family with a player piano at night. By day, he and Blue each gave half a dozen speeches to trade and civic groups, schools and clubs. Slowly, the two began to win popular support.

But Blue needed more than public approval. He also needed muscle and money from the city's business elite. So he urged the state medical society to invite six hundred of the city's civic, commercial, and professional leaders to a summit on the health crisis. A mass meeting planned for January 18 would galvanize the public, Blue was certain. But when the day came, it was a huge letdown.

Only sixty people showed up. The handful of physicians and public-spirited laymen looked lost in the vast hall. Despite the meager showing, those who attended resolved to grab the public by the lapels and draft civilians as active-duty soldiers in the war on rats. Mayor Taylor appointed a citizens' committee of twenty-five, led by Bank of California president Homer S. King and Chamber of Commerce president C. C. Moore. They formed the core of the Citizens' Health Committee, San Francisco's first grassroots army dedicated to fighting plague. The committee cranked out thousands of handbills. It issued a civic call to arms—summoning every profession, trade, church, temple, lodge, and ladies' club to rally for San Francisco's survival.

On January 28, hundreds of men in bowlers and fedoras came by buggy, cable car, and automobile to the granite-pillared Merchants' Exchange. The steel-framed neoclassical tower, designed by Willis Polk and Daniel Burnham, architect of New York City's Flatiron Building, had weathered the 1906 earthquake to become a symbol of survival. Its fifteenth floor held a cavernous mahogany ballroom and a curved bar as big as a whale where deal makers drank. On the exchange floor, Blue in uniform was flanked by Governor Gillett and Mayor Taylor.

No new human plague cases had developed in the last three weeks, Blue told them. But it was just a winter intermission. Rat infection levels had tripled since the fall. Without total eradication, the warm weather would rekindle the epidemic. If it flared as it did in the Orient, San Francisco would face massive mortality, quarantine, and economic ruin.

"Unless we obtain the support of the people," Blue said, "the task is hopeless." An optimist by nature, Blue had never uttered this word in public. *Hopeless.* He saw the effect on his listeners' faces; he was not displeased.[15]

There was another incentive, too. President Theodore Roosevelt was sending the Great White Fleet west, and it was due to arrive in San Francisco the first week in May. The flotilla of sixteen gleaming white-and-gold battleships of the Atlantic Fleet, with sixteen thousand sailors aboard, was circumnavigating the globe in a display of national pride and military might. The fleet gave San Francisco a chance to revel in patriotism and advertise its strategic advantages as a commercial and military port. It would show the world that, after earthquake and fire, the city of iron and gold was back. Its visit would boost business and real estate values. Even now, reception committees were wiring huge "Welcome" signs with strands of sparkling lights to gleam from every hilltop down to the bay. The pulses of hotel keepers, restaurateurs, and saloon owners quickened at the thought of so many visitors.

But to this city aquiver with anticipation, Blue delivered a sober warning: Admiral Robley D. Evans, commanding officer of the Atlantic Fleet, would ask about health conditions before landing. If the city couldn't guarantee it was plague-free, there would be trouble.[16] The fleet would be diverted to Seattle.

"Gentlemen, Admiral Evans is now *en voyage* to San Francisco with the fleet," he said. "When his ship anchors, the first thing he will do will be to send his senior medical officer to me to ask if it will be safe to land his officers and men. I very much hope that I can give you a clean bill of health so that he will not have to go up to Seattle without accepting the wonderful hospitality which you are preparing for him."

As Colby Rucker remembered it, "The silence was broken only by the busy click of business men's brains and in a moment all were busily scrambling for a seat on the sanitary bandwagon."[17] All at once, the business leaders had a goal and a deadline. They had three months to spruce up for the fleet or face cancellation of the most magnificent military pageant in city history. They hurled themselves into a frenzy of civic hygiene. They began to organize all the city's trades to hold meetings for their members. Corporate angels and individual donors heeded the call for funds to support the Citizens' Health Committee—including some donors who had been reluctant to recognize plague in the earlier outbreak. The city's commercial elite climbed aboard: Levi Strauss & Co., Southern Pacific Railroad, Wells Fargo & Co., Ghirardelli & Co., and the St. Francis and Fairmont Hotels. From utilities to railroads, banks to brewers, jeans makers to chocolatiers, they resolved to raise half a million dollars.[18]

Blue's next target was Butchertown. Every steak and chop, ham and sausage, came from the cattle yards, hog pens, and slaughterhouses set on the bay shore near Islais Creek channel. Butchertown was set far from the city center, so diners couldn't hear the bawling of doomed cattle or see the swill trough that produced their Sunday roast.

Butchertown's waterfront setting had long saved slaughterhouses the trouble and expense of incineration and scavenger services. Garbage was simply dumped at the water's edge and borne away by the tides. The cluster of wood warehouses and shacks stood on piers over the mud flats. As the tide rose, the bay rushed in under the shacks to sweep away the offal. At low tide, it was a groaning board; at high tide, it was a floating banquet for rats who swam up to dine.

"I'll never forget rowing down Islais Creek, and seeking the great, big, fat rats coming down at low tide to feed to the beach . . . millions of them," said one eyewitness, University of California physician Robert Langley Porter.[19]

Blue went to inspect Butchertown, his boots clumping along boardwalks rusty with oxidized blood. He sent men to document the innumerable sanitary violations. They didn't know where to start. Vats of viscera, barrels of intestines, stood waiting to be turned into sausage casings. Carcasses were dragged across soggy planks before being carved up and dressed for sale. Through gaps in the killing room floors, scraps fell to the marshland below. The rats fought fiercely over the spoils.

Blue was a plantation lad, reared in the country, steeped in the rural realities of farm life, so he was not squeamish. But what he saw in Butchertown was so foul that he judged his report unfit for public print—unless the butchers refused to cooperate. In that case, he would release the unsavory details to the newspapers, to be read by San Francisco shoppers and diners. Blue promised to withhold his exposé from the public only if the butchers cleaned house.

The city board of health launched hearings on Butchertown and its pork annex, Hogtown.[20] Some of the butchers tried to placate the federal doctors by staging a theatrical cleanup. Before a crowd of invited reporters, the butchers unleashed a gang of boys to beat on their wooden walls with sticks, driving gray herds of rats out into the open, where men poured boiling water on the animals. It was a grotesque show.

J. Nonnenman protested that his eponymous slaughterhouse was as clean as any and the victim of a city scheme to drive him out of business. Another competitor tried humor: His rats were the healthiest in the world, he said. The butchers' defense failed. Six slaughterhouses, several slovenly stables, and an incinerator were all condemned.[21]

Hearst's *Examiner* broke unwelcome news: Two percent of rats were now infected—clearly in the danger zone. "If the human population of the city were infected in the same proportion," the paper said, "there would today be 8,000 cases in San Francisco." It chided tight businessmen who groused about giving a few hundred or a thousand dollars to the plague campaign. The alternative, one month of quarantine, would cost over $20 million. "It's a question of our pockets, and perhaps our lives," the paper said.[22]

From the meat markets, Blue turned to the task of cleaning rats from the city's five thousand stables and countless chicken yards. In the early 1900s, San Franciscan householders insisted on their right to raise eggs at home and stable their own steeds. But the coops and stables provided nests of hay and spilled grain for rats, so Blue ordered them destroyed or rebuilt in rat-proof concrete.

Next, greengrocers along Front Street came under scrutiny. Fruit sellers and vegetable dealers were complacent about tossing banana peels, rotten apples, and wilted produce in the street. The produce district, as a consequence, was second only to Butchertown as a rodent restaurant. One of the city's largest markets yielded nine infected plague rats. When word got out about the discovery, women threatened to boycott the offending stores. Activists circulated "Don't patronize" lists of the worst offenders.

Women's clubs, enlisted by the Citizens' Health Committee, urged their members to reform their shopping, cooking, and cleaning habits. Patronize pristine food stores only, they argued, and boycott butchers and grocers whose premises are rat havens. Yellow placards were nailed on facades that failed inspection—followed by court summonses if the scofflaws didn't clean up.[23]

At the California Club on Clay Street, maidens and matrons in shirtwaists and smart hats listened as Colby Rucker gave a passionate sermon on the new religion of urban hygiene. Poison, trap, and starve them out was the new gospel. The federal plague officers won a host of female converts; the newspapers reveled in stories about the fair warriors in the plague fight.

"When you look in your garbage pails, ladies, think of me!" Colby Rucker said, deadpan.[24] Muffled laughter erupted. Rucker's speech took the starch out of science. He didn't mind being their poster boy for garbage. Let them laugh, as long as they made their homes plague-free.

Blue was more grateful for Colby's verbal panache than he ever could express to his face. "Dr. Rucker has been simply invaluable," he wrote in a letter to Kate on March 11, 1908. "I address audiences because I am compelled to; Rucker does it for the love of the thing. We call him 'garbage can Rucker' because that is his hobby."[25]

Rucker's antic speeches, a great favorite with the women's clubs, hid a tragic irony. While he was lecturing ladies on how to protect their families' health, his own wife, Annette, was losing hers. She was racked by bouts of coughing—asthma, he thought. He hired buggies to drive her to Ocean Beach so she could fill her lungs with healing drafts of sea air. It helped a little, but her doctor remained worried.

Though public oratory was still a new taste in his mouth, Blue endeavored to remake himself into an ardent preacher for public health. At a noontime meeting of two thousand Southern Pacific freight handlers in the basement of the Flood Building, Rupert Blue led a revival meeting on vermin.

"I intend to kill a rat or two myself tonight, and I want all of you to do the same. It is the noblest work you can do," he exhorted the men in a South Carolinian's best imitation of Teddy Roosevelt.[26] The rough and callused congregation grumbled skeptically at this doughty, drawling doctor. With his pomaded black hair, center part, and waxed mustache, he looked like a dandy in fatigues. But the railroad workers got the religion, especially after the city board of health boosted the bounty on rats from 10 cents to 25 cents for a male rat and 50 cents for a breeding female.

Blue, for his part, got more comfortable mounting the bully pulpit. And businesses dug deep, none deeper than the railroad. Southern Pacific executives pledged $30,000 to the plague fighters' war chest.

The evening of Valentine's Day, Blue ascended the altar to lecture the crowded congregation at the First Unitarian Church. His message was dire. The brawny Norway rat had overrun the city, he told them. Infection abounded as never before; the critical plague prevalence of 2 percent that he had endeavored to avoid was now a reality.[27]

The clergymen of the city started preaching plague eradication from every church pulpit and temple *bima* in town. They hit the streets to meet citizens in secular settings. "Cleanliness isn't next to Godliness," said Rabbi Jacob Voorsanger of Temple Emanu-El. "Cleanliness *is* Godliness."[28]

The Dutch-born rabbi's work for the plague campaign that year took an extra measure of fortitude. Just one month earlier, in January 1908, he had lost his daughter Rachel to tuberculosis.

The state board of health, under its president, Martin Regensburger, turned from a tool of plague denial to a firebrand for plague eradication. But like Rabbi Voorsanger, Regensburger had to pause from the plague campaign in January to bury his fourteen-year-old son, Harry, another tuberculosis sufferer.[29]

Annette Rucker's coughing grew deep and ragged. Her blooming cheeks grew hollow and wan. Still, she taught young Colby his letters and helped her husband's career by lunching with the Langley Porters and other members of the medical haut monde. Under her maiden name, Annette Guequierre, she wrote an essay about female plague warriors, saying San Francisco women "fought for the safety of their city as courageously as any Carthaginian mother of old."[30]

Blue and Rucker and their fellow officers delivered their speeches to clubwomen, shippers, teamsters, and builders. Mass meetings were convened from union halls and schoolhouses to the Dreamland Skating Rink.

"This city is in danger of a quarantine," Rucker told a skeptical crowd, "and I want you to understand that if a quarantine is placed on San Francisco, you people will imagine yourselves in the worst corner of hell. The days following the disaster of April 1906 will seem like a holiday picture compared to the days to be spent in a city quarantined for bubonic plague."[31]

One group of businessmen urged Blue to get it over with and declare a quarantine, if only to frighten the city's careless citizens into concerted action. "Friend, have you ever seen a city in quarantine?" Blue asked them gravely. "I have, and I love San Francisco too much to subject her to one."[32]

In six weeks, 162 meetings made believers of many. "It got so that a man could hardly go to church to pray, or into a cigar store to punch a slot machine that he did not hear something about rats and the plague," said local historian Frank Morton Todd.[33]

After years battling the city's inertia, Blue found this new momentum heady. For the first time, he sensed he had a shot at success. For the first time since the outbreak, San Franciscans were showing their mettle.

"My dear Mother," he wrote to Annie Maria in February 1908. "Times have been strenuous with me and the entire staff in this past month. I started an agitation on plague to arouse the citizens to a sense of their danger. This agitation has grown out of my control. The people are aroused. I am making [six] speeches a day. My staff is doing the same. I have received calls for addresses all over the state. I am about worn out but must keep the iron hot and the people demand that I must lead them." The city's spirit moved him.

"I thought New Orleans a heroic people," he wrote his mother, "but find that San Francisco is far greater."[34]

By now, Rucker's throat was so sore from speech making that his swollen uvula hung down the back of his throat. He begged a surgeon to trim the raw tissue. Dubious, the doctor warned he would lose his voice for days.

"Amputate it," Rucker persisted. He was so exhausted that the enforced silence seemed like a holiday. He spent a week whispering.[35]

Meanwhile, time had run out on City and County Hospital. The hospital was hopelessly overrun by rodents. In its waning days, Langley Porter and a fellow doctor had returned to the laboratory, where they witnessed the spectacle of rats eating old wound dressings.[36]

Now vacant of patients, the old clapboard hospital was demolished with dynamite, engines, and cables. Wards and dispensaries that had served poor San Franciscans since 1872 were reduced to a pile of plaster dust and jagged timbers. Then the rubble was torched, flames consuming the infected ruins under the watchful eyes and waiting hoses of the San Francisco Fire Department. After almost four decades of service, it had become one more rat refuge to be destroyed.[37]

Butchertown's foul shacks were put to the torch in the spring of 1908. But the fruit vendors, unlike the butchers, routed rats and transformed their businesses into sparkling showplaces. By the end of March 1908, the produce marketplace on Front Street was billed as "clean enough to eat off." To celebrate this achievement, five hundred citizens spread outdoor tables on Front Street, shaded by white canopies, garlanded with greenery, and set with cornucopias of apples, bananas, pineapples, and figs.

"Perhaps we have killed a million rats, but let us raise the score higher for the sake of San Francisco," said Mayor Taylor to rousing cheers. Purging plague rats was like evicting grafters from City Hall, he said.

Blue congratulated the greengrocers on their transformation. He tantalized his listeners with a vision of the city's future as a "health resort"—code words that spelled a tourist bonanza. Then it was Colby Rucker's turn. After praising the city fathers, he said, it's time to praise its mothers, the real force behind the cleanup.

"You know that if a woman tells a man to do something, he might as well do it gracefully. He's got to do it anyhow," Rucker said. A wave of applause rippled from gloved hands. The ladies gave three cheers for their champion. A brass band struck up "Home Sweet Home." As Rucker hopped down from the speaker's chair, his comrades paid tart homage to his speech with a gag gift of a dozen lemons.[38]

"Ain't It Awful?"

◈

"MY CAMPAIGN IS STILL in full blast," Blue wrote to his sister Kate Lilly in March 1908. A dozen medical officers and over 400 inspectors and laborers had carried on through the winter rains. But, he confided, "I fear an outbreak by the advent of dry weather."[1]

Worse, if the city's support flagged and his team couldn't finish the job right, he predicted the city would have "a plague scare every summer for the next 20 years."[2]

Barnstorming on the speaker's circuit, Blue was becoming a celebrity. Newspapers found that the courtly Carolinian made good copy. Pauline Jacobson, a reporter from the *San Francisco Bulletin*, came to the two-story Victorian house at 401 Fillmore Street seeking an interview.

Colby Rucker escorted Jacobson upstairs, where she saw a six-foot khaki-clad officer behind the desk. He stood and turned his blue gaze on her. If her prose is any indication, she swooned a little. Her story read:

A man of action rather than word—big, broad-shouldered, handsome, commanding in his plain brown officer's uniform. Yet modest and unassuming . . . a quaint drawling Southern wit and kindly sympathy always lurking in his eyes and under the slim mustache, one to inspire confidence and to make one feel if worse should come to worse, we would have a man at the helm.[3]

The reporter wanted to know why San Francisco was so resistant to public health measures and whether it was uniquely obstinate.

"I have encountered it before," Blue said. "In the South, fighting yellow fever, I have had to deal with a bristling shotgun quarantine." Here in San Francisco, he added smoothly, "it is your robust optimism."

Then Jacobson engaged Blue in a discussion of how Western civilization was blinded by hubris to the threat of disease. San Franciscans, she said, were far too smug about "our purifying tradewinds and our wonderful climate . . . our sanitation [and] our lovely porcelain bathtubs."[4]

"Plague is no respecter of individuals or places," Blue agreed, explaining that San Francisco was as liable to experience plague as India. "The Hindus have a religion which does not allow them to kill vermin of any kind," he added. "But if they have more vermin to transmit the plague, you have more garbage. You have more food for rats than any city I know of.

"Prejudice and ignorance may frustrate the best efforts of the sanitary authorities," he concluded. "I do not wish to alarm the people. I want them to get busy."

"Get busy" became the theme of the campaign. More glowing press followed the *Bulletin*'s profile. The *San Jose Mercury* sent its reporter Herbert Bashford to visit 401 Fillmore. Sparing no superlatives, he called Blue "the greatest sanitarian in the United States."[5]

The abundance of good press was irritating to some senior members of the medical profession. And no one was irked more than University of California medical school professor Robert Langley Porter. A distinguished pediatrician, infectious disease specialist, and neurologist, Langley Porter pitched in to help control plague on the city's waterfront. While he formed a warm bond with Colby Rucker—their two families dined and took carriage rides together—he developed an intense dislike for his commanding officer. "Rupert Blue was just a public relations man," he grumbled years later. "Colby Rucker was the fellow who really did the work."[6]

But Rucker was equally adept at orchestrating publicity for the plague campaign. He was Blue's disciple, spreading the gospel of urban hygiene. He helped write his speeches and articles. He walked to work with him, lunched with him, planned professional dinners, and drank with him. They dined with officer friends or local politicians at the city's Bohemian Club, the private preserve of politicians and tycoons, artists and writers. Public health officers weren't rich enough to be regular members. But as visiting officials, they were welcomed as guest members and even admitted to the club's extravagant costumed theatricals—called the "jinks"—at the Bohemian Grove in the redwoods north of town. Eating and drinking, singing songs or telling tales, the animated Colby tried to ease Blue's doubts and dark moods.

Blue was nearing exhaustion, and despite signs of progress, he had plenty to brood about. The rat eradication campaign was superficial. At street level, the city looked cleaner. But what went on beneath city streets? The subterranean life of rodents was a mystery to him. Where did they hide and migrate? Infected rats had been found in every part of town except the city's sparsely settled western neighborhoods, the Sunset and Richmond districts. Now that many of the rats were trapped, poisoned, and cemented out of homes, where would they go next? He had to find out.

That's when it hit him—colors. He would dye healthy white laboratory rats red, blue, or green, each color denoting a district. Then he would release the rats back into the sewers, in order to see where they popped up next. The scheme disclosed the animals' migratory routes and helped him guide exterminators about where to place the tons of rat bait they purchased every month.[7]

But Blue's rainbow rats provoked howls of derision in the press.

> *If you should see a tiny mouse*
> *Whose hide was salmon pink,*
> *Would you not join the temperance band,*
> *And blame it on the drink? . . .*
> *Fear not these harmless little things*
> *That scurry round and squeal;*
> *They're all in Dr. Blue's employ*
> *And all of them are real.*[8]

Clever as it was, the rainbow rats project didn't produce any breakthroughs for Blue. For the rats were so widespread that nothing but massive, citywide extermination would suffice.

Pulp satirists weren't Blue's only problem that spring of 1908. A delicate diplomatic problem arose at headquarters. A friend of President Roosevelt's, it seemed, had an interest in the Stearns Company, the manufacturer of Stearns' Electric Rat and Roach Paste, the same product that had accidentally poisoned San Francisco children. In the wake of this mishap, Blue had banned the use of the product as too dangerous. But now Wyman—who knew of the poisonings—wrote a letter asking Blue to review the merits of all products and forcefully promoted Stearns' Paste as worth another try.

Wyman, never prone to lavish praise of his officers, even sweetened this request with an unwonted compliment. "I have been intending to write you a personal letter, especially to express my gratification at the way things have been handled in San Francisco, but I have been so busy that I have been unable to get at it," he wrote.[9]

Would Blue choose science and safety or yield to pressure from the surgeon general? There was only one right answer. Blue steeled himself. The choice of rat bait was a city matter, he replied. (That wasn't strictly true. True, the city paid for the bait, but Blue got to pick his poison.) Pressure to funnel business to a presidential friend didn't come every day. However, when the safety of San Francisco's children was at stake, favoritism toward a hazardous product was out of the question. He turned Wyman and the favor-seeker down.

Now Blue began driving his rat catchers to kill more animals, the laboratory men to run more tests. Carroll Fox, with his black spade-shaped beard and meticulous scientific method, had been appointed to succeed Halstead Stansfield. Blue had tried to brace Stansfield up, but to no avail. Stansfield was mired in depression and undone by drink. Blue was a sanitarian, not a clergyman or counselor. He could only hope Stansfield would master his grief and return to the campaign.

But on the morning of Monday, April 13, Stansfield left his rooms at the Majestic Hotel on Sutter Street. He rode out to Sutro Forest, a eucalyptus grove on the flanks of Twin Peaks. He walked into the brush. From his coat, he withdrew a .38-caliber pistol, put it to his right temple, and squeezed. Two men hiking after dinner found his body in the brush.[10]

Blue assigned Colby Rucker the grim errand of claiming the corpse and attending the city inquest. Officially ruled a suicide, Stansfield's death drew an attack on the plague campaign by a popular journal of satire and political commentary called the *Wasp:*

A MAD SCIENTIST

Upon His Work Has Been Based the Fake Plague Panic in San Francisco. . . . Proofs of so-called plague in San Francisco rest entirely upon the bacteriological findings of the late Dr. Halstead A. Stansfield, who committed suicide on Monday April [13th], in the Sutro Forest. . . . The evidence was indisputable that Dr. Stansfield had been erratic for a long time and his melancholia [was] intensified by intemperance. Yet it is upon the scientific findings of this mentally unhinged specialist that Dr. Blue and his associate plague experts pronounced San Francisco as suffering from an epidemic.[11]

Blue had seen trouble coming. He had always worried that if Stansfield ended up in the drunk tank, he would bring scandal and discredit to the public health service. But this was worse than he'd feared. Stansfield was in the morgue. His tragedy, splashed across the press, now cast doubt upon the plague diagnosis. Blue gave laconic interviews, outlining the facts for the newspapers. If he felt guilt over his officer's death, he kept his own counsel.

Colby Rucker had seen Stansfield's sprees as the prelude to disintegration. Without blaming Blue directly, he privately deplored the public health service's failure to diagnose mental illness and offer help to its men. Elsewhere, an unstable officer was discovered playing Peeping Tom by beachside bathhouses. Later, he died in an insane asylum. Another officer lost his mind, after struggling to mesh three clashing sets of data. He wrote a confession and killed himself. Rucker faulted the service for failing to recognize when its own doctors were in distress.[12]

Despite the shock of Stansfield's death and the gleeful press frenzy, Blue had to marvel at how steadily his team carried on. They worked long hours. They created fresh strategies against the predatory rats. Their novel solutions saved lives.

Officer Richard Creel ran Plague District One, which encompassed Chinatown, from a small frame cottage in Portsmouth Square. One day he discovered rats scuttling beneath the plank floors. Creel thought back to his Missouri boyhood. He recalled his parents' tales of how local farmers had saved the harvest from rats by raising the corn bins onto stilts. Dr. Creel propped up his own office on stilts and evicted the vermin.

One night shortly afterward, Creel met Blue and another officer, Charles Vogel, for dinner at the Little St. Francis, where all three lived. Vogel was despairing over the persistent plague deaths in the Lobos Square refugee camp. The camp's 750 Red Cross cottages had been soaked with carbolic acid. But even after disinfection, the pestilent rats returned. Then Creel spoke up. He told his story of the corn farmers and his own success in outsmarting the predatory rats. Convinced, Blue ordered the cubelike cottages of Lobos Square to be mounted on stilts eighteen inches off the ground.[13]

After eighteen plague cases in Lobos Square, the disease simply ceased. Raising the frail shacks on poles placed them too high for rats to climb in and created a crawl space for cats and dogs to chase them out from under the cottage floors. "Rat-proofing by elevation," a country cure that saved the corn, now became an urban success story that saved lives.

As the inspectors soldiered on, condemning slovenly houses and sordid cafés, they risked the wrath of property owners. The owner of a greasy spoon cursed and swung a claret bottle at inspectors, while a gun-toting housewife railed at the "grafters."[14]

Entering suspected plague houses was also fraught with risk of disease. Before crossing the threshold, the inspectors unleashed guinea pigs, letting them run through the building as furry flea magnets. This technique—along with doses of antiserum—limited the risk of lethal bites.[15]

The *Chronicle* and the *Wasp* continued to print acid attacks on the plague campaign. *Chronicle* publisher Michael de Young changed the tenor of his campaign in the *Chronicle*. Now, instead of flatly branding the plague a fake, he refined his editorials, affecting a new tone of scientific skepticism about the link between plague and rat fleas. He ran guest columns by contrarian physicians who lent an air of authority to de Young's plague denial. Blue warned Washington that de Young's pseudoscientific articles threatened to erode support of the public and of City Hall at a critical moment.[16]

This time, however, the state and county medical societies leapt to Blue's defense. Without naming names, they blasted certain newspapers as "a disgrace to reputable Journalism, a menace to Public Health and safety and an outrage upon the cities of their publication."[17]

The *Chronicle* backed off, and City Hall stood firm.

The rat work ground on. For the week that ended May 4, Blue quickly scanned the figures: 20,907 houses inspected, 190,104 bits of poisoned bait placed, 4,063 rats trapped, 2,518 rats collected from bounty hunters, and 691 rats found dead. Of these, the men tested 2,952 rats for bubonic plague bacteria. Sixteen animals were infected. The prevalence of infection was subsiding—from the flashpoint of 2 percent, it was down to 1.2 percent—better, but not good enough.

San Francisco was visibly cleaner by May. The produce markets were pristine. Butchertown was rebuilding. Though some work remained, the trends were so favorable that Surgeon General Wyman called on President Theodore Roosevelt to deliver the good news for which the city had been waiting. It was safe for the Great White Fleet to land inside the Golden Gate.

Half a million people stood on the hills and headlands that May morning. Cannon concussions split the air and thudded in the chests of the onlookers as the flotilla of white-and-gold warships glided through the Golden Gate. From the ship decks, the men could hear the cheers and see the fluttering of thousands of tiny flags, antlike in their agitation, on the hillsides. The city was awash with joy. Businesses were ecstatic.

A bisque-complexioned Gibson girl in a pale gown adorns a commemorative poster. Poised gracefully on a giant bar of Pears' soap, she is shown gazing out over the bay, waving her handkerchief at the fleet. The Great White Fleet and Pears' soap, said the ad: "Two of the world's most valued necessities to protect our women and keep them happy."[18]

On the eve of his fortieth birthday, Blue seemed immune to the thrill. Perhaps seeing the city's excitement over the navy aroused some buried boyhood rivalry with Victor. For certain the municipal holiday stole attention away from his duties at the lab. "Owing to the enthusiasm over the presence of the Fleet, things are very quiet at the present time," he wrote Surgeon General Wyman. "As soon as this temporary excitement is over, I will resume the educational campaign."[19]

Blue was itching to unveil a new "stereopticon" lecture series that had dazzled his audience at a recent state medical convention in San Diego. While he lectured, the device could display a picture of a warty-tailed *Rattus norvegicus,* then magically dissolve the image into a picture of a flea. He could make a slide of a patient with classic buboes dissolve into a microscopic mugshot of *Bacillus pestis.* He wanted Colby Rucker to take the stereopticon lecture on tour to the American Medical Association in Chicago.

It would take more than magic lantern slides to reclaim the public's attention after the splash made by the Great White Fleet. Next to all that glamour, San Francisco's zest for the plague campaign slumped, in a kind of morning-after languor. "The people, I fear, are lapsing into an apathetic state again," Blue reported to the surgeon general. He added bitterly, "The occurrence of a case at this time would tone them up a bit."[20]

Of course, Blue wasn't hoping for another human casualty. But the persistence of infected rats told him that pockets of plague still smoldered underground. Such a reservoir of germs could fuel outbreaks indefinitely. As long as danger persisted, his work wasn't done. If he couldn't keep the public engaged, he would fail. He'd been battling plague for eight years now. If San Francisco could stay the course for another eight months, he could finish the job and leave behind him a healthy city.

Blue realized by his birthday on May 30 that San Francisco hadn't suffered a human plague case in months. This wasn't a guarantee of anything, as recent reports from Sydney, Australia, had shown. There, plague came roaring back after a seven-month respite. Here, summer was approaching, high season for fleas, when plague cases peak. Blue wrote to Washington to head off the city's efforts to win a premature clean bill of health for the city.

"I fear," said Blue, "that August and September will see a re-crudescence of the disease."[21] Recrudescence—the ugliest word in the public health lexicon—means an epidemic outbreak after a latent spell. Like a war that flares up after a seeming peace, it humbles the soldier who has underestimated the enemy.

Somebody was bound to jump the gun. On Sunday, June 14, 1908, it happened: *The New York Times* declared victory against plague in the city of San Francisco.

> Under the superintendence of Rupert Blue of the Public Health and Marine Hospital Service, a war of extermination was waged. . . . When these Pied Pipers finished their work, there were no rats left in San Francisco, and as a consequence the plague has been effectually [sic] stamped out.[22]

No one from the *Times* had bothered to interview Blue. Had they done so, they would have learned that, far from being over, the rat war had captured 4,929 rats that very week and 5,000 the week before—including several plague carriers.

Blue spent a lot of time that season setting the record straight, countering press reports that were too optimistic or pessimistic. Progress was undeniable now, but a premature pullout would ensure a return of the disease. He warned his family that he wouldn't return home for awhile.

"My work may be satisfactorily completed by late fall, and I may then return to the 'Effete East' in quest of other adventures," he wrote his sister Kate in late June. "On the other hand, the disease may reappear and hold me in the 'Golden West' for six months longer." Moreover, he allowed, the social opportunities for a single officer in the West were tempting.

"Tell Mother that I am still single but that the 'fair heads' out here are very hard to resist," said the forty-year-old bachelor. "That sometimes in the course of human events, I extricate myself with difficulty and reluctance."[23]

The daily grind of the rat campaign was wearing down Colby

Rucker. In early July, he took to bed with chest pains. Although he was only thirty-two, he felt sure that he had heart disease and resorted to a then-popular cardiac compound: digitalis mixed with arsenic. The pills left him anxious and depressed.

On July 4th, Rupert Blue called on his second in command at home. The two men sat together out on the front porch, chatting and chewing over politics in the public health service's commissioned corps. Blue and Colby's five-year-old son observed the holiday by lighting caps together. "The quietest Fourth I have ever known," Rucker reflected.[24]

Three days later, the Great White Fleet weighed anchor and took its leave of the city. Rucker, feeling stronger, took a carriage to the Presidio to watch the flotilla depart, savoring the sight of each white-and-gold vessel dipping its flag in farewell as it left the Golden Gate.[25]

In a real sense, the city owed the visit of the fleet to the plague doctors, just as the doctors owed their success to the fleet. But Blue could not enjoy the spectacle. He was stewing over the fact that his annual report on the plague war wasn't ready. Surgeon General Wyman, a martinet with a penchant for perfect paperwork, would surely send a reprimand. Rucker interpreted Blue's preoccupation as a personal reproach. He felt Blue didn't value the fact that he'd worked every day through his illness. Struggling through his own chest pain and Annette's coughing, Rucker tried his best to keep up with the mounting workload.

Rucker also took pains to try to humor his moody boss. The men often lunched together at the Bohemian Club, the Fairmont, or the Majestic Hotel, sometimes playing dominoes afterward. They dined at Coppa's, a Latin Quarter bistro offering crusty loaves and rough red wine, fresh pasta, and Chicken Portola for under a dollar. Long a favorite of hungry artists, Coppa's walls were chalked with murals of nude gamboling nymphs and gods, which the upright Rucker found mildly scandalous. Champagne suppers at the club or officers' dinners in the leather banquettes at Blanco's often lasted till two A.M., leaving a four-hour nap before he had to rouse himself and get to the office on Fillmore. Annette wasn't pleased about these escapades.

On his wedding anniversary, Rucker took a rare day off, hired a buggy, and drove with Annette to Lake Merced for a picnic celebrating their six years together. They had a rustic feast, strolled the lakeside, made peace. But Rucker's diary entries betray the strain of struggling to please those closest to his heart.

"I did not sleep well through worry about Annette and why R.B. has been so offish of late," he wrote. "Possibly thinks I am trying to get ahead of him which is not true. . . . Perhaps I am over sensitive."[26]

The day after Colby and Annette's anniversary picnic, Blue acted cool toward his second in command, as if to reprimand him for having taken his anniversary off. A workhorse who led by example, Blue wanted his men to work weekends and evenings, giving them just a half-day break on federal holidays. As a divorced officer of forty, he had no family to come home to; thus all days were alike to him. His world was the lab; his universe, the city and its epidemic. Rucker, on the other hand, had made a world with the wife he adored and their child. He radiated fulfillment, in painful contrast with Blue's solitude. Rucker, an only child, had produced a son and heir. Blue, one of eight siblings, was childless and seemed more and more likely to remain so. Rucker was a constant reminder of Blue's own failure at love.

Tension between the officers was exacerbated by fiscal strain. City leaders, their treasury exhausted, begged the public health service to stay the course. Mayor Edward Taylor appealed to President Theodore Roosevelt to keep federal funds flowing. "All the money and energy expended so far will count for naught unless the campaign is continued with unabated vigor until the last traces of the rat infection has [sic] disappeared," Mayor Taylor said.[27] Blue backed his appeal.

Just when San Francisco seemed on the verge of being controlled, an unforeseen tragedy struck in the East Bay.

Joe Farias, the seven-year-old son of a Portuguese rancher near Concord in Contra Costa County, fell sick with symptoms that were by now too familiar: fever and tender glands under his arm. The public health doctors would immediately have recognized the peril, had they known. But before they even heard of the case, the boy was dead. The microscopic evidence pointed to plague.

Two more East Bay victims followed that same week. Rumors from the local ranchers told of rats, staggering around as if dazed or drunk, reeling in slow motion, and so helpless that the ranchers killed them easily with a stick.

Blue dispatched his most trusted officer by ferry, train, and buggy into the tawny grasslands to solve the mystery. Despite his grim errand, Colby Rucker was dazzled by the rural bounty. "This is a rich, fine, warm country, full of olive oil, fruit, wine and wheat," he wrote in his diary. "A campaign against squirrels must be waged if we are not to leave a frightful heritage to posterity."[28]

Within a week after the death of Joe Farias, Rucker zeroed in on a site heavily infested with rodents, just a mile and a half from the Farias family ranch. Rucker found dead rats at the site and brought one grim trophy back to the city in a glass jar. McCoy tested the animal. It had the plague.

Tightening the noose, the trappers next closed in on the ranch itself. There, on August 5, they found something unexpected: a sick and listless ground squirrel. Tests on its body confirmed that the animal was suffering from the same *Bacillus pestis* as the city and country rats.[29]

It was a breakthrough. In Asia, scientists had long known that plague could jump between city rats and wild mammals like marmots. But here was the first proof that, through the exchange of fleas between rats and squirrels, American plague had infected western wildlife. And it had happened with disturbing speed. Now they had a new animal host, and the perimeter of plague was flung wide open.

The discovery, Blue wrote Washington, was "perhaps the first demonstration of the occurrence in nature of bubonic plague in the ground squirrel (*Citellus beecheyi*) of California." As the animals inhabited the whole state, he added, "the discovery has caused considerable apprehension."[30]

In San Francisco, the team was tackling another question. Back at 401 Fillmore Street, Blue ordered the rat trappers to bring rats back alive. Baskets of the wriggling prey were emptied into glass jars with chloroform-soaked gauze.

Once the scrambling rats slowed in their struggle and grew still in their death sleep, district officers combed their fur for fleas—by now also dead. They put the fleas from each rat into glass bottles filled with alcohol. Each bottle was labeled with the date, type of rat, and the district from which it was captured. The flea wranglers then sent their catch to 401 Fillmore Street.

Colby Rucker pored over flea anatomy with a sense of wonder. He marveled that the flea has the largest, most powerful hind legs of any creature its size, enabling it to jump five hundred times its length—a feat equal to a human vaulting over a skyscraper of almost two hundred stories. The flea, he asserted, was responsible for more annual deaths than any monstrous reptile or carnivore in nature.

For an essay entitled "The Wicked Flea," Rucker peered through the microscope and discovered that the sesame seed–size specks were armed with armadillolike plates, triangular slashing weapons, two lances, and a stiletto with which they pierced their victims' skin and sucked their blood. Rucker also studied the mating habits of fleas; during their courtship, he watched as the "lordly" males sat back in a passive role, while the females engaged in a frenetic dance of seduction. After coupling, the female laid a clutch of waxy ovoid eggs that, over her lifetime, could produce up to five hundred hungry hatchlings.[31]

Even less savory were the fleas' dining habits. With horrid fascination, Rucker observed the suckling parasites in action with his colleague George McCoy. McCoy rolled up his sleeves and, holding the fleas under inverted test tubes, allowed the insects to feed on his bare arms. The men found that, after eating, the flea left a deposit on the skin of its victim. When the victim scratched, this deposit got rubbed into the skin. Scratching helped to inoculate the bacteria with deadly efficiency. The lab fleas, fortunately, were healthy.

Years later, scientists would discover that the material injected by a flea into its victim was actually blood from a previous bite. After several feedings, these previous blood meals collected in the flea's foregut, welling up like heartburn, to be injected into the bite wound on the next victim's skin.[32]

But Rucker and McCoy's colleague, Carroll Fox, made a curious discovery: In San Francisco, the prevalent flea species was not the Oriental or Indian rat flea, *Pulex cheopis*. While there were a few of those in the city, the main flea species on the Golden Gate was the northern European rat flea, *Ceratophyllus fasciatus*.[33] Beyond being of academic interest to entomologists, what possible difference could that make?

Plenty, as it turned out.

For San Francisco had had a stroke of dumb luck. The plague flea's key trait wasn't its armor or its stiletto, but its gut. Although Fox didn't appreciate the significance of his findings at the time, scientists now know that the Asian flea *cheopis* grows a basket of spines in its belly. Inside that basket, a clot of blood collects, forming a potent ball of plague germs. The clot also blocks new blood meals from reaching the flea's stomach, so it begins to starve. That makes the ravenous flea attack more aggressively, biting any warm-blooded animal that crosses its path. Finally, its frenzied sucking dislodges the ball of germ-laden blood. It is, in effect, this flea heartburn that delivers a lethal dose of plague into its hapless human host.

Fasciatus, the Frisco flea, has a foregut without that spiny basket. So while it is capable of transmitting plague, each injection delivers a less potent—that is, less infectious—dose of the germs. *Cheopis,* the lethal flea, visited San Francisco, but it remained in the minority. Had it taken over to become the dominant species on the Pacific coast, the toll of the sick and the dead might have been far higher.

Although he didn't know it at the time, Fox's finding about local flea species provided a clue to later scientists as to why San Francisco's plague claimed hundreds, rather than thousands, of casualties. The plague germs were as deadly, the rats as numerous, the fleas as hungry. The only difference may have been a quirk of flea anatomy.

With so much energy funneled into flea studies in the San Francisco laboratory, Indian summer commenced with little fanfare. Warm, sunstruck, and treacherous, September 1908 was ripe for a resurgence of human plague. Blue remained edgy and watchful.

Without warning, word of a setback came from the southern tip of the state. Health officers in Los Angeles, four hundred miles to the south, had a sick ten-year-old boy on their hands. Doderick Mulholland, who lived in the Elysian Park neighborhood of Los Angeles, fell suddenly ill with a fever and tender knobs sprouting from his glands. A dead squirrel was found near his house. The Mulholland boy was biopsied and tested positive for plague. The animal, too, harbored the bacteria. But the young boy lived. To everyone's relief, his case remained an isolated one. Plague did not establish a foothold in Los Angeles—not yet, anyway.

Managing operations on three fronts, Blue decided that a frontal attack on the squirrels was the fastest way to purge the countryside. But squirrels are wary and lightning-fast, nearly impossible to bait and trap. He wrote to Washington, asking $1.50 a day to rent rifles and buy ammunition. Once more, he tripped over red tape. Washington reproached Blue for sloppy form in making his request, denying him funds.

Colby Rucker had greater woes. One evening, after giving a speech in San Jose, Rucker dined with Annette's physician. The doctor frankly confided his fears about her cough. "In truth it worries me too," Rucker wrote in his diary. "But I don't know what to do."[34]

As Annette lay pale and fatigued, her son, Colby, tried to beguile her with a popular new song on the player piano. He inserted the roll, and out pealed the song "Glow, Little Glowworm." Annette smiled wanly, but a nurse hired to tend her hushed the boy. "Let the boy play," Annette implored. He was allowed to finish the tune, but he never touched the instrument again, forever hating the song that couldn't make his mother well.[35]

With rumors of many squirrels dying, and Washington dragging its feet, Rucker bought himself a $9 rifle and some maps. He packed up his family and ferried them to the East Bay. The warm, dry weather might be good for Annette's lungs, he thought. He staged a buggy excursion to the East Bay peak of Mt. Diablo, with watermelon picnics by the roadside. Annette gained a bit of strength. When Rucker returned to San Francisco, he marked a birthday and found tufts of gray sprouting over his ears. He was thirty-three years old.[36]

Meanwhile, the epidemic retreated in San Francisco. The month of September, which had seen fifty-five cases the previous year, ended without a single new case.

By October 1908, Blue counted a lapse of eight months since the last case of human plague in San Francisco. From May 1907 to February 1908, plague had sickened 160 San Franciscans and killed 77 of them. It was a broader and swifter outbreak, more democratic in its choice of victims, but less deadly than the smoldering plague of 1900. That earlier episode in Chinatown took a narrower aim on the Chinese, and case for case, it was far more lethal, with an official count of 121 sick and 113 dead. However, given the suspicion by many white doctors that the community had hidden some of its sick and the dead, the true total would never be known.

The reported death rate fell from 93 percent in 1900 to less than 50 percent in 1908, due in part to earlier diagnosis and better supportive care. The absence of racial scapegoating, and Blue's conduct of the second campaign, left people less fearful, less prone to conceal their sickness, and more willing to see a doctor.[37] However, it's also possible that a certain number of undiscovered cases in the China-town outbreak actually survived plague; had these been diagnosed and counted, they might have lowered the death rate. No one will ever know; the true toll remains part of the last century's secrets.

But Blue now began quietly trimming his city crew, hoping it was safe to do so. At the same time, he was uneasy about the situation in the East Bay. He renewed his demands that Washington fund a corps of squirrel trappers to pursue the infection spreading in the country-side.

Back in town, Colby Rucker was worn out by work and worry over Annette's lungs. "Foggy bad morning," he noted in his diary. "Walked home in the rain. Spent the evening at home feeling rotten blue."[38]

An unnerving discovery in October 1908 shook the team's confi-dence. In a warehouse strewn with discarded fruit and nut shells, a rat was lured by the scent. Up the elevator shaft to the fifth floor it scuttled. A trap sprang shut. Back at 401 Fillmore Street, the men chloroformed, skinned, tacked, and dissected the rat. They prepared the tests. They hoped for a negative result. No luck. The rat was teeming with plague. It was the first plague rat found in eighty-five days. As Blue had warned so often, they couldn't discount the stealth or the staying power of an entrenched foe.

There would be no victory just yet. Colby Rucker wrote of the re-versal in his diary that day. In an aside, he jotted a bit of 1908 slang: "Ain't it awful, Mabel?"[39]

The Pied Piper

THE CITY'S DANGEROUS decade seemed to be ending. After trapping the plague rat inside the California warehouse, inspectors tore the place apart, looking for stragglers. It turned out to be the last of its infected breed.

The *San Francisco Call* hailed Rupert Blue as a hero and a "modern Pied Piper who can charm rats out of their holes with a whistle."[1]

In the Robert Browning verse "The Pied Piper of Hamelin," the town failed to pay the piper his fee for getting rid of rats, and instead paid with the loss of its children. San Francisco, another heedless town, also paid a fearful price for its negligence: 281 sick and 190 dead of plague.[2]

Blue must have felt satisfied as he and Rucker surveyed the statistics of their public health campaign. More than 11,000 houses had been disinfected. Over 250,000 square feet of Victorian boardwalks had been replaced with concrete sidewalks. Over 6 million square feet of homes, shops, and stables were now girded with rat-proof cement floors.[3]

More stupefying were the rat statistics. Blue's brigades had set out over 10 million pieces of bait. More than 350,000 rats had been trapped, killed, and collected from bounty hunters. Over 154,000 animals had undergone bacteriologic tests at the Fillmore Street rattery. Most of the vermin, however, were trapped far below the city streets. All told, the total kill was estimated at more than 2 million rats—*five times the human population of the city.*

For months, San Franciscans saw great gray rafts of rat cadavers wash out of the sewers and into the bay, floating on the waves and bobbing against the rocks, until at last the tide swept them out to sea.

Gradually, the currents and the brisk salt winds swept away the stench of chemicals and rat kill. The city's natural perfume of brine and sun, eucalyptus and woodsmoke, sourdough and coffee, returned. The campaign continued to deliver other dividends, too. Not just plague, but *all* infectious diseases started to subside. Clean homes and shops, remodeled sewers, pure food and water—together, these improvements curbed a host of diseases from typhoid to diphtheria.

Amid the city's return to health, its rebuilt downtown area sparkled in the fall and winter of 1908. In two years since the earthquake, twenty-five new skyscrapers thrust up from the flattened city center. Nine reconstructed landmarks, including the Palace Hotel and the Chronicle Building, reclaimed their spots on the skyline.

A new Chinatown arose from the ruins like an electrified phoenix. Old wooden shops were replaced by illuminated pagodas that bathed the district in peacock hues. Old-timers along *Do bahn gai,* Dupont Street, shook their heads in dismay over this transformation. But the tourists returned in droves to stroll, sip tea, and buy curios. The city's sense of fun, which years of suffering had all but eclipsed, came roaring back.

Buffalo Bill's Wild West Show brought its gaudy spectacle to Market Street in the fall of 1908. Nearing his eightieth birthday, the old showman Colonal William F. Cody shook his grizzled locks in wonder at the city's rebirth. "San Francisco," he said, "why she's all right. The earthquake and the fire were blessings in disguise. They have made your city the most modern in the world. If it were not for the fatalities incurred, a shake-down would be a good thing for all big cities."[4]

Nobody, not even Blue, would have claimed that plague was good for San Francisco, but the eradication program doubtless left it a healthier city.

Headlines on Thanksgiving 1908 proclaimed the long-awaited recovery:

CLEAN BILL OF HEALTH GIVEN
SAN FRANCISCO: SURGEON
GENERAL WYMAN REPORTS
PACIFIC COAST STATES
FREE FROM PLAGUE[5]

Blue couldn't celebrate right away. Just as plague left, the winter of 1909 blew a ferocious influenza into town. The past year, he'd escaped. This year, Blue caught the virus he called "my old and unterrified enemy." Sicker than he'd been in years, Blue was confined to bed at the St. Francis and nursed for three days by hotel housekeepers and waiters. He was so weak that he apologized in his next letter to his sister Kate because his filigreed penmanship wasn't up to par. "My hand," he explained, "is somewhat shaky."[6] But he rebounded in time to receive the thanks of the city.

On the late winter night of March 31, 1909, San Francisco spread a feast on Nob Hill to honor the Pied Piper of Marion and his men. Nine years since the death of the first victim, Wong Chut King, and one year since the last plague case, the ordeal was over.

That evening, Blue and his officers shed their khakis for evening dress, straightened one another's bow ties, and piled into cars and buggies, bound for the Fairmont Hotel. Once past the white stone-pillared portico, they traversed the gilt-and-marble lobby, en route to a balconied banquet hall. There four hundred of the city's elite paid $7.50 to dine with the health officers whose mission they had scorned in 1900.

A vast expanse of black tails and broad white shirtfronts met their eyes. Photographers took flash pictures that burst like sheet lightning over the hall, blanching faces and making the celebrants blink. The white-napped tables boasted hothouse flowers and menu cards engraved with the evening's bill of fare. Each course was a corny conceit on the theme of plague. Oysters came first, but not Blue Points, the menu said, because "he's been giving them to us for years." Next came a course of striped bass, released from quarantine. Vegetables were prepared from the city's pristine produce district. For dessert, ice cream was molded in the shape of a mousetrap. Punch was poured into tin tankards that looked like garbage cans, with the slogan "Keep the lid on." Lurking inside each drink was a toy rat favor.

Governor Gillett, Mayor Taylor, and merchant-activists applauded the release of new health figures showing that the federal cleanup had not only quelled bubonic plague, but slashed the rate of other communicable diseases like diphtheria and scarlet fever by 75 percent.

Blue looked across the crowd. There were the city's prosperous and powerful, recent converts to the cause of public health. Then there were his men: his loyal aide, Colby Rucker; and thin, bespectacled George McCoy and black-bearded Carroll Fox, the flea wranglers. There were old faces from a decade ago, such as H. A. L. Ryfkogel, the crippled pathologist who had helped Blue and who was spied on, fired, and denied back pay for his trouble.

In keeping with early 1900s social customs, dinner was a masculine affair. Not invited to dine, the women of the plague campaign were cloistered in a gallery high above to hear the speeches.

When Blue was called to the dais, an ovation roared for five minutes. His old shyness flooded back, and he flushed scarlet. "It's difficult to say much when the heart is full," he began. "I feel as if I were one of California's adopted sons." He saluted the local men—the inspectors and rat catchers—whom he called "the brawn and sinew" of his campaign.

"San Francisco has set an example," he said. "It behooves all seaport cities to look to their sanitary defenses, for there is where the disease enters. San Francisco has fought her battle, and as one of you, I am proud of the victory she has gained."[7]

Mayor Taylor presented Blue with a gold pocket watch. The heavy gold disk sprang open to reveal an inscription engraved within: "To Rupert Blue, Passed Assistant Surgeon U.S.P.H. & M.H.S., from the citizens of San Francisco in grateful recognition for his services to the city while in command of the sanitary campaign of 1908." The mayor then pinned medals on fourteen public health service officers.

A bass chorus of hurrahs erupted again, joined by cheers from the women in the gallery. As Colby Rucker had often reminded them, the city's cure was their triumph, too.

With Hearst's usual flair, the *Examiner*'s editorial page declared the next morning, April 1, that the dinner presaged a golden age of health in the twentieth century. "Man's conquest of disease," it said, "is certain."

But it wasn't really over. The plague that had menaced the city still thrived in the hills and grasslands just east of the bay. As soon as the winter rains subsided, and the mud-softened country roads were firm enough for buggy wheels, Blue sent his forces rolling into Contra Costa County with camping equipment and War Department tents. By striking early, he hoped to prevent a crop of human cases during the summer. He wanted Colby Rucker to lead the charge on the squirrel plague again. Surgeon General Wyman had other ideas. He planned on transferring Rucker up north to Seattle. But Blue begged the surgeon general to reconsider. Rucker was the most seasoned plague warrior he had. And there was the matter of Annette.

By now, her diagnosis was unavoidable.

"Mrs. Rucker, I regret to state, has pulmonary tuberculosis," said Blue in a handwritten postscript to Wyman. She was feverish now and bedridden. "The doctor does not desire that any special provision be made for him on this account but does not wish to have to take her to Seattle as the climate is not good there. R.B."[8]

Surgeon General Wyman relented and let Colby Rucker stay with the campaign. When the spring sun dried the roads, Rucker returned to the East Bay hills leading a handful of men armed with sacks of poisoned wheat.

But during the years of delay, the infected squirrels had dispersed widely, migrating over a vast swath of north central California. By mid-1909, plague had invaded 1,500 square miles of suburban and rural terrain—more than thirty times the space it had occupied in the forty-nine-square-mile city of San Francisco.

Surveying this new infected zone, Rucker underwent "the most terrifying and grizzly experience of [his] life." One Sunday morning, he and two colleagues struck out to explore some infected burrows with a load of guinea pigs. To test for infected fleas, the scientists tied a string to a guinea pig's leg and lowered it into a suspect burrow as a flea magnet. Then they would fish out the guinea pig, comb it for insects, and analyze them for plague. That day, however, they needed no guinea pig. From several paces away, they beheld a graveyard of squirrel skulls around an abandoned burrow, out of which swarmed a strangely pale cloud—fleas.

Three feet above its opening, the famished fleas attacked the men. "Is your life insurance paid up?" one colleague joked nervously. Rucker fought the urge to run away. Now the fleas jumped and wriggled under his clothes, biting furiously. When the work was done, Rucker returned to his hotel and stripped off his fatigues to find his skin as mottled with bites as if he'd had a full-blown case of measles.

An entomologist on the team assured him the fleas were hatchlings, too young to have sucked the blood of plague squirrels. Rucker thought grimly of all the corpses he had seen, bulbous and stained with the blue-black tokens of plague. "I knew just what they would find on my body at post-mortem," he said. But the entomologist was right: The beige hatchlings were baby fleas. All three men escaped unscathed.[9]

The squirrel plague worsened inexorably, as did Annette's health.

"It is impossible for me to be in so many places at one time," Rucker confessed, and asked for an assistant. "Mrs. Rucker's condition is very critical," he said. "It is only a matter of time until I shall be obliged to ask for a leave on her account, and I would very much regret seeing my work pass into untrained hands."[10]

Rucker stayed with the campaign. To carry him on his rural surveys, he got a noisy Buick roadster, which lurched over country roads. He left the ailing Annette in camp with a trained nurse. But fearing his son might contract tuberculosis if left by his mother's side, Rucker took the boy on his road trips, tying him into the car with an improvised seat belt to keep him from bouncing out over the country roads.[11]

Rucker found that about 1.2 percent of the animals were infected already. Burrow to burrow, the infected squirrels were crossing the coastal hills, migrating eastward toward the Sierra Nevada. Surgeon General Walter Wyman asked his officers to map the territory, so Rucker sketched the state of California and shaded the plague zone with black ink.

Studying the plague map, Surgeon General Wyman finally beheld the results of years of red tape and delay: The lands now inhabited by wildlife infected by the plague spread out to cover a vast area that resembled a giant letter *P*.[12] *P* for "plague."

Digging in for a protracted battle against the squirrel plague in 1909 and 1910, Blue closed up the old Victorian headquarters on

Fillmore and moved his office to San Francisco's rebuilt downtown area. On New Montgomery Street, he outfitted his office with unusually posh appointments: a swivel chair, a rolltop desk, and a $35 rug from W. & J. Sloane. He now divided his time between the city and travels abroad as the government's epidemic expert-at-large. When Chile suffered a plague outbreak in 1910, he sailed down to the coastal town of Iquique, where one hundred patients languished in a rat-infested lazaretto. When Panama and Hawaii were menaced by yellow fever mosquitoes, Blue advised the canal zone and the islands on epidemic control.

While Blue was on assignment overseas, Rucker remained in Berkeley, where his wife, Annette, died of tuberculosis in May 1910. Rucker and his son, Colby, transported her body to Milwaukee for burial. He remained in the Midwest for a year.[13]

In November 1911, Surgeon General Walter Wyman was shaving around his trademark walrus mustache when his razor slipped. The sixty-three-year-old Wyman was a diabetic, so a simple shaving nick posed a special threat. His diabetes-damaged vascular system couldn't fight off the infection that grew in the flesh wound. Gangrene set in. With no antibiotics to fend off the infection, toxicity streamed from the wound into his bloodstream. Helpless against the overwhelming sepsis, Wyman fell into a coma from which he never recovered. He died, leaving the nation's public health service without a leader.

As President William Howard Taft launched a search for Wyman's successor, candidates sprang up from the ranks of senior officers to jockey for the job. The front-runner was Joseph White, Blue's onetime commander and critic in the plague war. It was White who in 1901 initially disparaged the younger man as genial but inert, devoid of the energy and tact required of a plague commander. In the end, the two fought both plague and yellow fever side by side. Now they found themselves rivals for the public health service's top post.

Joe White had seniority, and conventional wisdom gave him the inside track to become the next surgeon general. Rupert Blue was clearly his junior, but his success in San Francisco had raised his public profile and cachet as a man of action.

Colby Rucker, after a rough year in Milwaukee, returned to the public health service and began to lobby for Blue for surgeon general. Realizing he hadn't actually consulted Blue about this, he sent a telegram in Hawaii: "Wyman dead. Have entered you in race. Too late [to] back out now."

Blue wired back: "Go to it."[14]

The campaign intensified and press speculation mounted. President Taft teased reporters a bit by saying they could pick their favorite color. One way or another, he hinted, the new surgeon general would be Dr. White or Dr. Blue. But the president didn't deny he was favoring Blue.[15]

Blue was summoned to Washington. He kept his family in the dark about his rising fortunes. "Let us hope that the best man wins, for we need a Moses to lead us out of the wilderness of political intrigue," Blue wrote to Kate just before Christmas. He coyly added that he expected to get "orders at any moment to get me hence to the alfalfa patch faraway beyond the Rocky Mountains."[16]

But another tour of duty in the West wasn't his destiny. On January 5, 1912, President Taft flouted convention and sent to the Senate his nomination of Rupert Lee Blue for surgeon general. Blue was confirmed, amid a groundswell of support for his record as an epidemic fighter.

The forty-six-year-old South Carolinian "was promoted over the heads of many older men," commented the *Medical Times* of New York. "President Taft, recognizing the fact that the important public health service must be directed by the wisest and sanest and most skillful man in the corps, forgot the bugbear of precedence and nominated the best man."[17]

Blue was moved his fellow officers thought him worthy of holding the highest office in the corps. His joy was incomplete, however. His mother, Annie Maria Blue, died that autumn in Marion, months before her youngest son became the highest physician in the land.

Blue's first task as surgeon general was anything but exalted. He had to inspect the health of government buildings—a job he'd handled for Wyman back in 1906. Little had changed: Unsanitary cuspidors steeped the State Department in the scent of tobacco juice. Rats overran the Department of Justice.[18] Toilets and drinking water were petri dishes for germs. Blue focused on the common drinking cup, a foul feature of many public facilities, and began replacing it with fountains, a simple change that slashed the cases of contagious disease.

Blue sketched for his family the life of a presidential appointee: the long days and nights at his desk, marked by moments of ceremony, such as donning his best bib and tucker to wish Happy New Year to the outgoing President Taft on January 1, 1913. He rarely made it home to Marion to see his sisters. His brother Victor and sister-in-law Nellie sent him a gift of Christmas cake, its taste recalling "the days of long ago when I had no responsibilities and few troubles." He worked through the holiday, confessing, "All seasons and days are alike to me. . . ."[19] Now that he was deskbound, his once athletic frame thickened.

As surgeon general, Blue broadened his agenda to embrace a revolutionary new concept: national health insurance. Although it was as radical a notion then as now, national health insurance drew support from the American Medical Association (AMA). Good health is a right, Blue insisted. Promoting it was, in his view, the surest way to enhance the moral stature and happiness of a people. Moreover, he argued, it was a good investment, and every dollar spent on public health would be returned a hundredfold.

"Public health is a public utility," he said in a speech before a 1913 convention of life insurance executives. "It is the great glory of the period in which we live that we have recognized our responsibility as our brothers' keeper."[20]

At this moment, all Blue's instincts as a physician and a southern populist merged and flowered. In the middle of his tenure as surgeon general, Blue was elected president of the American Medical Association, becoming the only doctor ever to hold the two posts simultaneously. He made national health insurance the centerpiece of his administration.

"There are unmistakable signs that health insurance will constitute the next great step in social legislation," he said. "The next great step in social legislation" became a rallying cry of the national health movement. One of its key supporting groups, the American Association for Labor Legislation, emblazoned Blue's phrase across its stationery. But national health insurance found more support among public health professionals than private physicians.[21] It withered before it could take root. Nonetheless, in 1915, the AMA gave Blue its Gold Medal Award, as the member who had done the most to promote the health and well-being of humanity.

Renominated in 1916 by President Woodrow Wilson, Blue planned an attack on diseases of the poor like hookworm and trachoma, a major cause of blindness. But soon his domestic agenda yielded to a global imperative: preparing the country for World War I. The public health service was temporarily made a branch of the military it had emulated for so long, with its uniforms and martial style. Blue readied the country's doctors and hospitals to receive flood tides of casualties. But neither his upbringing as a soldier's son nor his years in the public health service prepared him for reports of the carnage in trenches across the Atlantic.

"I had never thought that I would live to see such a colossal war that is prevailing in Europe," he wrote to his sister. "It is simply barbarous."[22]

In 1918, in the wake of war came a lethal epidemic of influenza. Among the casualties was a veteran of the San Francisco plague campaign. Donald Currie, posted to Boston in 1918 just as the epidemic hit the eastern seaboard, contracted the flu virus and died.[23]

Influenza wasn't the only wartime epidemic. Soldiers came home bearing another scar of their service abroad: venereal disease. In an era when polite society shunned the topic of social diseases, Blue launched a vigorous VD prevention program aimed at young men. He also attended and admired a play in Washington entitled *The Aftermath*, about the scars left by VD. Struck by the power of drama to enlighten people about public health, he urged President Wilson to see the play. Hoping for a presidential boost to his prevention campaign, Blue wrote to Wilson's secretary, urging the theater outing. Coaxing reluctant politicians to embrace controversial health campaigns was an art Blue had refined in San Francisco. But this time, he failed. At the bottom of Blue's invitation, the commander in chief jotted his regrets: "Sorry, but I cannot. W.W."[24]

After two terms as surgeon general, Blue now began to lose favor in Washington. The massive World War I–era conversion of hospitals into veterans facilities—ordered by Congress, but without adequate funding—stressed local governments and strained political relations.

VA hospitals were Blue's responsibility, and he took the heat for their troubled conversion. Meanwhile, cabinet members seeking political favors decided to appoint as their next surgeon general a candidate from Virginia. They chose Hugh Cumming, a tall, aristocratic Virginian with suave political instincts and none of Blue's World War I–era political baggage. At fifty-two Blue was out of office, his ambitious dreams of national health insurance dashed.[25]

At a career juncture where many prominent men play golf and pen their memoirs, Blue resumed active duty in the public health service and refused to step down until he reached retirement age. Accepting the lower rank of assistant surgeon general, Blue tackled domestic disease outbreaks and traveled to Europe as U.S. delegate to international health congresses, including the League of Nations. In Geneva, he addressed such challenges as worldwide opium addiction and the need to create a standard medical lexicon to aid in global disease tracking.

In 1923, Blue received a distinction beyond the dreams of a lad from Catfish Creek. France decorated him as a Chevalier de la Légion d'Honneur.

"You will recall that as a boy I admired the First Napoleon perhaps more than any figure in history, and that I never tired of reading his life and of his deeds as a soldier and statesman," he wrote to his sister Kate. "I never thought then that I would ever receive, much less deserve, the decoration which he bestowed upon his officers and men, that of the Chevalier of the Legion of Honor. . . . I wear the ribbon in the lapels of all my coats."[26] Finally, he had a decoration that shone as brightly as the military hardware adorning the chest of his elder brother Victor.

But Blue's fall from political favor left a wound that never healed. In 1924, during one long night of drinking and dredging up the past with his old friend Colby Rucker, the pain and bile welled up. He denounced his rivals as "snakes" and "damned skunks." Even Rucker, whose career had flourished under Blue's successor, received an undeserved share of rebuke. Blue called him "a God-damn apostate."[27]

It was too much. Rucker left his mentor alone that night, and the two men remained estranged for half a dozen years.

Their long silence ended when Rucker—ever the peacemaker—

sent Blue a New Year's card in 1930. Blue responded gratefully. But only a few months after this tentative thaw in their relations, Colby Rucker died. Having survived encounters with rats, fleas, and mosquitoes, Rucker fell victim to a sting by a yellow jacket on a golf course near New Orleans. The sting became infected with streptococcus, and in the era before antibiotics, the complication proved fatal. He was fifty-four years old.[28]

Blue survived his protégé, living as an old bachelor at the Hotel Benedick at 1808 "Eye" Street off Farragut Square in Washington, D.C. He continued to send money faithfully to his unmarried sisters, Kate and Henriet. After his brother Victor died of heart disease, he remained an attentive uncle to Victor's sons, John Stuart and Victor Jr. The boys fretted over their uncle's solitary life.[29]

Blue wasn't quite as solitary as they feared. Having long resisted the "fair heads" of San Francisco, he was at last won over by a dark-eyed Washington socialite. Lillian de Sanchez Latour, widow of the Guatemalan ambassador to Washington, had reigned over Embassy Row parties in the 1920s. Now she became Blue's companion in his autumn years. So discreet was their friendship, it came to light only when the U.S. government took the unusual step of sending Mme. Latour a formal letter usually reserved for next of kin.[30]

It was a letter of condolence.

After a lifetime of vanquishing exotic epidemics like yellow fever and plague, Blue fell victim to the same fate as his father and brother: heart disease. Advancing arteriosclerosis sent him to seek treatment in Baltimore, then he headed home to South Carolina.

Just one month shy of his eightieth birthday, in a hospital in Charleston, Blue's heart gave out. Borne home to the Presbyterian church in Marion, he was carried to the town graveyard hung with Spanish moss and lulled by the song of the cicadas. A church quartet sang the old hymn "Lead Kindly Light."[31] He was lowered into a grave surrounded by those of his family and by the multitudes of marble angels and stone garlands in the old southern cemetery.

His headstone, a monolith of gray granite, towers over those of his sisters Kate and Henriette. Austere in the South Carolina sun, it bears only one ornament: the public health service emblem he wore on his belt buckle as a green recruit—the caduceus of the messenger god Mercury, patron of commerce. But the design, like Blue's career, bears more than a passing resemblance to the staff of Aesculapius, ancient healer, who raised the dead and riled the gods.

"His work for humanity took him to many lands," reads the inscription, "but he came home to sleep his long last sleep."

Epilogue

◈

No monument stands in San Francisco to mark the city's plague ordeal and the public health warriors who fought against it. The epidemic, once extinguished, was all but forgotten.

Joseph Kinyoun, the bacteriologist and quarantine officer who diagnosed San Francisco's plague, was chased out of town as an archenemy of the people. As a scientist, he was undone by mercenary politicians, who bartered the city's health for trade. He was a victim of official denial and protectionism. But his character, in turn, fed the city's animus. He was proud, isolated, dismissive of the very plague patients who most needed his help. Clashing with the Chinese and pouring fuel on the city's anger, he was, in his own view, at war with everyone. Kinyoun's quarantines and travel restrictions against Asians, while supported by his superiors, were crude and discriminatory tools. Moreover, we now know that, even if the courts had not overturned them, such measures would not have stopped bubonic plague. Wounded and uncomprehending, Kinyoun quit San Francisco, and shortly afterward, the public health service. His career on the national stage was over, and its premature end was a reminder that science without compassion is a dry and punitive discipline.

After leaving San Francisco in 1901 at age forty, Kinyoun returned to the East and worked as director of a company making vaccines and antitoxins, as a professor of bacteriology and pathology at the George Washington University School of Medicine, and as the city bacteriologist of Washington, D.C. During World War I, he served the U.S. Army as an expert epidemiologist. Not long after the armistice, however, Kinyoun developed an aggressive lymphoma of his neck. In 1919 at age fifty-eight, he died.[1]

History has been kinder to Kinyoun than his contemporaries were. For his founding role in the National Hygienic Laboratory, forerunner of the National Institutes of Health (NIH), he is posthumously recognized as the first director of the NIH. It was the work of his youth—applying the powerful tools of bacteriology to the diagnosis of infectious disease—that survives him, untainted by the political and racial poison that infected so many people in 1900.

Rupert Blue, who leapt from San Francisco to the surgeon generalcy, fared far better. To some degree, history favored his endeavors. Just when he took command of the situation in San Francisco, medical science finally grasped the facts about the transmission of bubonic plague. And it was Blue who put those findings into practice in San Francisco. Once rat fleas were identified as the primary culprits, Blue could spare people the ruinous consequences of quarantine, and focus on killing rats.

The personae of Kinyoun and Blue are a study in the making or unmaking of an effective public health leader. Kinyoun had the science and the intellect, but he lacked human relations skills as well as a vision of what public health could bring to suffering populations. Whatever his private feelings about race, Blue did not antagonize San Francisco's long-suffering minority community. And despite his professed phobia for public speaking, Blue possessed the polish and charm to engage the public, to persuade, to educate, to galvanize change in the field of public health. More than that, he had a populist vision of harnessing public health, not just to lock out epidemics at the border, but to alleviate suffering and improve the life of the people.[2]

However honeyed his style, his leadership wouldn't have worked had not Blue, the pugilist, known when it was time to take off his gloves. As historian Guenter Risse has said, "Friendly persuasion was reinforced with intimidation." It was only when he threatened the feckless city with loss of the Great White Fleet that Blue "fully engaged the powers of his office" as commander of the plague campaign.[3]

As the sanitarian who liberated San Francisco from bubonic plague in 1908, Blue gained a reputation for the kind of vigorous epidemiology the country needed. He served as the country's surgeon general from 1912 to 1920, a period when world conflict and vast migrations of soldiers once more carried diseases around the globe. During World War I, Blue fought the twin epidemics of influenza and venereal disease. Although the AMA in 1915 named him the doctor who did the most good for humanity, his legacy was damaged by global events over which he had little control. Saddled with that nightmare of all reformers—an underfunded congressional mandate— he struggled to convert hospitals nationwide into veterans medical centers with too little staff and money to do the job. Had he been a tougher politician, he might have managed it, but it's likely no administrator could have met all the demands of postwar civilian and military health. Under such pressure, Blue's dream of a third term devoted to national health insurance died. His goals of mandating universal milk pasteurization and a network of child health clinics were dashed as well. By 1920, Blue was out, his public health vision outdated and undone by a welter of political forces. He remained in the public health service as an assistant surgeon general, serving in domestic plague outbreaks and in international health conferences.

Despite years spent purging plague on the San Francisco Bay, Blue had failed in all attempts to push his victory beyond the county line. For years, he had warned Washington about the danger of plague spreading to squirrels in the countryside. He had implored Washington for men, tents, rifles, and traps to rout the rural infestation. But his requests were deferred or denied. By the time he got approval to send a force into the East Bay, it was too late. Plague had spread to wildlife over thousands of square miles of California hills and grasslands.

It didn't stop at the East Bay hills, but spread eastward, over the Sierra Nevada mountains and into the Rocky Mountains. In each zone, the fleas found a new host animal, jumping from rats to ground squirrels, then to the golden-mantled squirrels of the Sierras, then to chipmunks and prairie dogs who inhabit villages of burrows throughout the Southwest. Plague's natural reservoir has always been rodents, and it found a home in the wildlife of the American Southwest, where it still smolders a century later.

Today, pockets of wild plague are scattered over vast territories around the globe. Colby Rucker's 1909 plague map, with its P-shaped stain over California, has grown into a thick band of plague that covers the western third of the United States from the Rockies to the Pacific. Around the world, plague is scattered widely across Eurasia, Africa, and the Americas. Over the last five decades, the World Health Organization has monitored plague reports from thirty-eight countries, including notification of over eighty thousand cases and almost seven thousand deaths. Seven countries experience plague cases almost every year: Brazil, Congo, Madagascar, Myanmar, Peru, Vietnam, and the United States.[4]

Modern plague scientists from the U.S. Centers for Disease Control and Prevention (CDC)—men and women who are heirs to Rupert Blue—run a surveillance station in Fort Collins, Colorado. While the disease is considered too deeply embedded in the wild to be eradicated, the CDC and state health departments monitor wildlife, control fleas, and report to the WHO. When plague levels rise dangerously high, they post warnings to protect hikers and campers and sometimes even close state parks until the danger subsides. Warning signs showing a squirrel inside a red circle with a diagonal slash are a common sight in parklands throughout the West.

Such vigilance doesn't prevent about a dozen people in the United States from contracting bubonic plague every year. Hunters, trappers, campers, and country dwellers are at the greatest risk. The expansion of residential development into the high deserts and foothills of New Mexico, Arizona, Colorado, and Utah brings people closer to plague country. Cats and dogs exploring infected burrows can pick up fleas and become a link between infected wild rodents and people. From 1977 though 1998, twenty-three people contracted plague from sick cats. Five of them died, casualties of misdiagnosis or delayed treatment.[5]

For patients today, modern antibiotics render the plague far less deadly. A course of intravenous streptomycin or other antibiotic offers most people a ready cure. But its efficacy depends on a swift diagnosis and timely treatment. Doctors in the Southwest are acutely aware of what a sudden attack of swollen glands and fever can portend. Such knowledge has saved scores of people in recent years. One of them was Debra Welsh.

Right before New Year's Day 2000, the forty-three-year-old woman, who lives in the country north of Albuquerque, New Mexico, noticed that her house was invaded by little drunken, wobbly mice. She caught the mice in her hand, holding them with a paper towel. She flushed them down the toilet and washed her hands with antibacterial soap. Later, odd symptoms emerged.

A swollen lymph node appeared. The chills began. Intense aches and back pain hinted of something more grave. Following admission to St. Joseph's Hospital, she was diagnosed with bubonic plague. A course of twenty-first-century antibiotics saved her from a medieval fate.[6]

A century after its discovery, untreated plague remains one of the most deadly diseases known to humankind. Without treatment, the mortality of bubonic plague ranges from 50 to 70 percent. When untreated plague spreads to the lungs or bloodstream—as pneumonic or septicemic plague—the mortality rises to nearly 100 percent.

Since plague is so lethal, San Francisco was lucky to have only 280 reported cases. Some people might wonder whether this represented a real epidemic. Kenneth Gage of the Centers for Disease Control and Prevention says the answer is yes. An epidemic is defined as any increase over the normal, baseline incidence of a disease. Before 1900, plague had no normal incidence in the Unites States. The San Francisco plague cases represented the first known outbreak in the continental United States. From that outbreak, plague established a foothold across the western states. Today, despite preventive vaccines and antibiotics, plague occurs in roughly a dozen people a year. Even forty cases of bubonic plague in any twenty-first-century American city would be considered an epidemic and an emergency. So 280 confirmed cases and 172 deaths certainly qualifies.

"San Francisco was clearly an epidemic," confirms Gage—no relative of the old California governor. "We would go crazy if we had that number of cases right now."[7]

Gage is a plague expert with the CDC in Fort Collins, Colorado. As an authority on the odd parasitic relationship between rat and flea, Gage says the San Francisco outbreak could have killed many more if it weren't for that odd quirk of anatomy in the flea's gizzard. He is among those who believe that the 1894 plague pandemic killed millions in Asia partly because its carrier was the Oriental rat flea, with its spiny foregut. Dr. Gage believes San Francisco was spared a similar fate because most of the local fleas lacked the anatomy of a killer.

All the other ingredients for an epidemic of devastating mortality were in place: the same bubonic plague germ, a massive population of rats, and a populace numbed by racism, ignorance, greed, and protectionism. A mote inside a speck of an insect saved the Barbary Coast from the fate of Florence or London.

People might wonder if San Francisco had a milder strain of plague bacteria. But Gage says this is unlikely. The strain covering the western United States today, which emanated from 1900 San Francisco, is the same one that savaged Asia and spread around the globe during the pandemic of 1894. Even more powerful evidence of this shared strain is the fact that those who did contract plague in San Francisco died with breathtaking speed. The mortality of the first plague outbreak in Chinatown was 93 percent. In the second citywide outbreak in 1907, the mortality rate fell to under 50 percent, thanks to faster diagnosis, hospitalization, and treatment with Yersin's antiserum. Such treatment, though primitive by today's standards and lacking in curative antibiotic drugs, would have included fluids, fever medication, and nursing care. It may have helped save patients' lives, or at least eased their deaths.

The decade of the Barbary plague, 1900–1909, was a transitional moment in history between Victorian and modern San Francisco. Many of its landmarks have been destroyed by earthquake or razed by subsequent development. The corner of Dupont (today's Grant Avenue) and Jackson Street, the site of the Globe Hotel, where Wong Chut King died, is today occupied by a glass-fronted retail bank. Where the Japanese brothel once stood, small trading companies and clothing stores rub elbows with souvenir and herbalist shops. The Merchant Street laboratory was leveled by the 1906 earthquake, but the alley remains as a passage between Chinatown and the skyline-piercing tower of the Transamerica Pyramid. Portsmouth Square, once dotted with quarantine tents, is a park once more where children play and aged Chinese do their morning tai chi exercises.

The Victorian house at 401 Fillmore Street that was home to the plague lab and rattery is now gone, replaced by a bland stucco apartment. Lobos Square, where the plague attacked eighteen refugees in their earthquake shelters, is now a park called Moscone Playground, just a block from the marina and yacht harbor. But the century-old Merchants' Exchange on California Street is intact; strollers can still walk inside the building where Rupert Blue rallied the citizens and transformed their apathy into activism.

Angel Island is now a state park. Nothing remains of Kinyoun's 1900 quarantine station at Hospital Cove, now Ayala Cove. Immigrants' detention barracks, opened in 1910, are now a museum where poems carved in Chinese characters on the walls give mute testimony to the pain of exclusion. The smell of disinfectant baths is today replaced by the scent of barbecue. Boats arrive to disgorge not waves of immigrants, but waves of picnickers who come for a day in the sun.

San Francisco's epidemic response, though slow to arouse, served the city well almost a century later in 1981, when acquired immunodeficiency syndrome struck its homosexual community. In the early days of the AIDS epidemic, when denial or discrimination clouded the country's vision, San Francisco was a model of swift and compassionate care. Today, as other epidemics strike, stricken countries must sometimes learn all over again that the politics of denial, commercial protectionism, and discrimination too often trump science and sound medical judgment. Mad cow disease, or bovine spongiform encephalopathy, a brain-wasting disorder, ravaged British cattle herds in the 1980s and 1990s. The human form of the disease, called variant Creutzfeld-Jakob disease, has so far lethally infected 125 people in the process. Might this tragedy have been avoided if government and industry has acted sooner? Denial, protectionism, and the search for scapegoats arise when epidemics strike. The politics of 1900 San Francisco, far from being an anomaly, simply forshadowed the dynamics of epidemics to come.

By now, a sophisticated public knows that germs don't respect national boundaries. Yet ironically, when plague struck India in 1994, Americans eyed their international airports with terror. What if a person, sick with the highly contagious pneumonic form, had boarded a plane in Bombay or Delhi and landed in New York? Those who were the most afraid didn't know plague was already deeply imbedded in the landscape of the American West. Borders that were porous a century ago are even less substantial today in an age of jet travel. Disease fighters at CDC have even less time to prepare than they had in the era of travel by steamship.

The eradication or control of many infectious diseases from smallpox to polio has led us, we're often told, to a false sense of security. In September 2001, the arrival of anthrax spores in letters awakened the world to the reality that old diseases may return as tools of terror.

Erosion of the public health system left the country vulnerable, just as these diseases come out of retirement. Whether they are in the hands of domestic murderers, stateless terror cells, or large state-funded weapons programs, this threat requires the same preparedness for massive outbreaks as the country faced in centuries past.

In a haunting counterpoint to Blue's struggle to subdue plague, several countries of the world have studied the germ as a candidate for biological weapons. As early as the fourteenth century, Tatar soldiers hurled plague-infected corpses over town walls in the present-day Crimea. In World War II, the Japanese refined germ warfare a bit, by raising infected rats and fleas in grain-filled bathtubs, and sifting the lethal insects over unsuspecting people in China. After decades of official denial, the Tokyo District Court in August 2002 acknowledged that the attacks took place, in a reversal reported by the world's press.

During the Cold War, the United States explored making plague weapons, but was thwarted when the germ cultures lost virulence over time in the test tube.[8] The project was abandoned, but not without exacting a price. In 1959, a young chemist who was analyzing plague at the U.S. Army's laboratory in Fort Detrick, Maryland, was swept by chills and fever, vomiting, and a bloody cough. Despite having taken the vaccine and booster shots, he was saved only by massive doses of streptomycin. Narrowly surviving pneumonic plague, he suffered liver damage from his ordeal. Three years later, a veteran microbiologist at Fort Detrick's British counterpart in Porton Down, England, was less fortunate. While studying Y. *pestis* for defensive purposes, he contracted pneumonic plague and perished in a Salisbury hospital. After an investigation, his death was ruled a "medical misadventure."[9]

Both the United States and England abandoned their biological weapons research decades ago, and signed the Biological Weapons

Convention, banning germ warfare in 1975. However, the former Soviet Union continued its massive, covert bioweapons program until 1992. While debriefing defectors, Westerners learned for the first time of Soviet ambitions to create the deadliest of plague weapons— along with anthrax, smallpox, and other scourges. Unlike Japan's primitive rain of fleas on Manchuria during World War II, the Russians improved the hardiness of the plague bacterium, which it codenamed "L1." At its weapons plant in the city of Kirov, it maintained a quota of twenty tons of pure plague in its arsenal.[10]

Defectors such as Kenneth Alibek worry that the specter of plague as a doomsday weapon has secretly survived the public dismantling of the Soviet bioweapons industry. However, the threat has also given new impetus to ongoing scientific initiatives to analyze and understand the genetic blueprint of *Y. pestis.* In one breakthrough, announced just three weeks after the terror attacks of September 11 on the World Trade Center and the Pentagon, British researchers deciphered the complete genome of plague. The British Ministry of Defense is developing a new vaccine to prevent plague outright. American researchers are devising fast DNA fingerprinting systems to speed detection of the organism—whether it occurs naturally or arises at the hands of terrorists. French scientists are bringing into focus the special "virulence genes," which give plague a lethal edge over its ancestor *Yersinia pseudotuberculosis.*[11]

For plague doctors, the days before Paul-Louis Simond's flea discovery were like the days before Walter Reed discovered the role of mosquitoes in yellow fever.

"We were fighting in the dark," Blue said.[12]

Through his tenure as surgeon general and afterward, Rupert Blue revisited his years as a plague fighter. And sometimes they revisited him. Ragtag men would appear at his Washington office without an appointment, startling his secretary.

"Just dropped by to visit with Dr. Blue for a minute," announced the veterans of Blue's old rat brigades.[13]

Ushered into Blue's office, they saw a figure thicker about the waist, his boxer's chest now avalanched into a paunch that strained his vest and watch fob. Gray at the temples, he'd kept his trademark mustache. Blue welcomed the frayed visitors to reminisce a moment about the days of the quarter bounty and the rainbow rats.

Blue never lost his appetite for fieldwork—even after his tenure as surgeon general was over. He happily got back into harness to travel west and confront his old nemesis, the rat, when a plague outbreak claimed thirty victims in Los Angeles in 1924. He urged that the country maintain a standing force of public health officers ready to take the field to fight outbreaks at a moment's notice, as he had done throughout his career.

He often received letters from a public curious about the modern toll of an ancient scourge. One of them was from Alda Will, a woman in Coronado, California, who wrote the surgeon general seeking advice for a friend who had survived bubonic plague. She asked what lingering aftereffects her friend might suffer.

Dear Madam, Blue cautioned, the scourge of bubonic plague leaves "severe traces" on the human heart, and it may never be the same.[14]

Acknowledgments

AS A MEDICAL REPORTER covering epidemics from plague to AIDS, I had read and reread Daniel Defoe's *A Journal of the Plague Year,* for insight into the human dynamics of epidemic, and how fear drives people to folly. In 1994, just as I began a new assignment writing *The Wall Street Journal*'s health column, the plague resurfaced half a world away in India. The 1994 outbreak unreeled before Western eyes like a febrile nightmare: photos of masked Indian doctors tending the sick and the dead. The outbreak conjured up images of ailing jet travelers landing in New York or Los Angeles. My editors requested a column on the Indian outbreak. I wrote about how the U.S. Centers for Disease Control and Prevention surveillance teams were monitoring airports to prevent the epidemic from being imported. The CDC experts were alert to the threat of travel-borne disease, but mystified by the panic. Plague, they said, is already endemic in the wildlife of the western United States. What seemed like an exotic foreign scourge was, in fact, already at home on these shores. How plague came to America was a story I wanted to tell.

But reconstructing the history of a smoldering ten-year plague required help from many hands. Early in my research I benefited from reading the scholarly analysis of medical historian Guenter Risse of the University of California at San Francisco. Dr. Risse's 1992 article in the *Bulletin of the History of Medicine,* " 'A Long Pull, a Strong Pull, and All Together,' " opened my eyes to the political dynamics at work in quelling the outbreak, as well as to the wealth of primary source material documenting the episode. Moses Grossman, retired chief of pediatrics at San Francisco General Hospital, who has treated plague in children, offered early encouragement in the research. Scholars of the city's past, Gladys Hansen and Charles Fracchia of the San Francisco Museum and Historical Society, graciously shared their expertise. Susan Haas of the Society of California Pioneers guided me through her group's photo archives.

Special thanks are due to John Parascandola, U.S. Public Health Service historian, who was a generous guide to his field, sharing documents, insights, and interpretation. Like Chaucer's scholar, "gladly wolde he lerne, and gladly teche."

I spent a week happily plundering the documents at the National Archives and Records Administration in College Park, Maryland, with the assistance of ace archivist Marjorie Ciarlante, who met me with a hand truck the size of a Volkswagen bug, piled with boxes from NARA's Records Group 90, Central File (1897–1923). Inside lay the history of the U.S. Public Health Service plague fighters in century-old letters, autopsy reports, and telegrams that were crisp and tobacco-hued with age. Thanks are also due the staff of NARA's facility in San Bruno, California, where documents on the Angel Island Quarantine Station and 1906 earthquake are housed. I am grateful to Stephen Greenberg, Elizabeth Tunis, and all the staffers at the National Library of Medicine in Bethesda, Maryland, for help in researching the papers of Joseph J. Kinyoun, and for photographs and other documents.

At the University of California at Berkeley, I benefited from the rich holdings of the Bancroft Library and the East Asian Library. Special thanks go to librarian Wei-Chi Poon, who patiently checked out reel after reel of the century-old Chinatown newspaper on microfilm. My appreciation goes to Professor Charles McClain of Berkeley's Boalt Hall School of Law for his analysis of the clash between public health and civil rights. The San Francisco Public Library's San Francisco History Center was a haven for documentary and photographic research. Thanks go to Tom Carey and Pat Akre and their colleagues.

Unlocking the secrets of turn-of-the-century Chinatown culture would have been impossible without the help of my translator, Sister Prisca Hui, Roman Catholic nun and experienced translator. She interpreted scores of articles from the Chinatown daily newspaper, *Chung Sai Yat Po,* guiding me with humor and zest through the linguistic subtleties of the immigrant community on "Gold Mountain." I am indebted to many scholars of San Francisco's Chinatown for helpful discussions, including Him Mark Lai, the Reverend Harry Chuck, James Chin of the Chinese Consolidated Benevolent Society, Professor Judy Yung of the University of California at Santa Cruz, and the staff of the Chinese American Historical Society in San Francisco.

Plague scientists from the U.S. Centers for Disease Control and Prevention in Fort Collins, Colorado—Drs. Kenneth Gage, David Dennis, and May Chu—shared all they know about plague, from rats to fleas to human victims. The plague laboratory chief of the Pasteur Institute in Paris, Elisabeth Carniel, shared stories of venturing into plague zones from Vietnam to Madagascar—while pregnant and unvaccinated.

I am indebted to the people of Marion, South Carolina, for graciously tolerating a Yankee reporter who came to town in hot pursuit of the ghost of their native son Rupert Blue. The hospitality of Tom Griggs, cultural guidance of Tommy Lett, and the social history provided by Mmes. Elizabeth McIntyre, Suzanne Gasque, and Lucia Atkinson, along with Judge T. Carroll Atkinson III, imparted understanding and flavor to my project. Special thanks to Robert McCollum, owner of Bluefields plantation, for letting me tour the house where Rupert Blue grew up.

My friend Mary Christine Kartman deserves thanks for helping with the quest for information on Lillian Latour, Rupert Blue's vivacious, jet-eyed autumnal romance, and for braving the handwritten notes of the historian Bess Furman, and locating a plague journal on microfilm.

It is a challenge to do research on a hermetic hero who "never complains, never explains" and rarely divulges his personal life in his professional milieu. For such was the persona of Rupert Blue. After much searching, I located descendants of the Blue family—Eleanor Stuart Blue of Washington, D.C., and J. Michael Hughes of Jacksonville, Florida. Ms. Blue, the great-niece of Rupert Blue, cordially shared memories and memorabilia of her great-uncle, including the gold watch given him by the city of San Francisco. Mr. Hughes, Blue's great-nephew, was patient with my persistent inquiries, and finally located in his attic a cache of personal letters of Rupert Blue's covering almost a half century of his extraordinary career. Boundless gratitude to both for entrusting me with family treasures.

I owe similar thanks to Colby Buxton Rucker of Arnold, Maryland, for entrusting me with diaries and other writings—both unpublished and published—of his grandfather William Colby Rucker's, who was, for almost forty years, Rupert Blue's sidekick in battles against bubonic plague and yellow fever. Dr. Rucker was Dr. Blue's Boswell, and was as transparent and emotive as his boss was opaque and stoic. His account of the plague campaign opened a window on Blue's character.

Heartfelt thanks to Estella Cox Collins of Durham, N.C., the great niece of Dr. Joseph Kinyoun, for her generous permission to quote from the letters of Dr. Kinyoun's mother, Mrs. John Hendricks Kinyoun, contained in the family papers collection at Duke University.

My deep gratitude also goes to Joan Procter of Sausalito, Calif., for giving her family's permission to reproduce the photograph of the steamship *Australia* taken by her grandfather John W. Procter and archived at the San Francisco Maritime National Historical Park.

None of my research and writing would have been possible without the support of many editors and colleagues at *The Wall Street Journal,* including managing editor Paul Steiger and deputy managing editor Daniel Hertzberg. Thanks to bureau chiefs Gabriella Stern, Michael Waldholz, and Elyse Tanouye, and to deputy bureau chiefs Ron Winslow and Bob McGough. In San Francisco, thanks are due many colleagues, including Steve Yoder, Carrie Dolan, Ann Grimes, and Sharon Massey.

My agent, Henry Dunow, is a champion for his swift and intuitive grasp of my project from early days, and for prodding me to mine those mountains of inert documents until I found the human pulse of my story.

Nobody could be more fortunate than to have Random House editor in chief Ann Godoff as mentor and guide, grooming my book from the mortifying mechanics of a first draft to the finished manuscript. Her zest for everything from the scientific arcana to the dynamics of narrative drive opened my eyes to the storyteller's art. I'm grateful for the energy of Sunshine Lucas, and the early enthusiasm of editors David Ebershoff and Courtney Hodell of the Modern Library. Affectionate appreciation goes to Random House senior editor Ileene Smith and her staff, especially Robin Rolewicz, for adopting the project at a critical moment. Thanks to Todd Doughty, Liz Fogarty, and Dennis Ambrose for their help.

Every researcher stands on the shoulders of giants, and I found a dozen willing to put aside their professional duties to read my manuscript: U.S. Public Health Service historian John Parascandola, plague scientists Drs. David Dennis, Ken Gage, and May Chu, Dr. Moses Grossman, Chinatown historian Him Mark Lai, San Francisco historians Gladys Hansen and Charles Fracchia, medical historian Guenter B. Risse, law professor Charles McClain of U.C. Berkeley, and law and public health scholar James G. Hodge of Johns Hopkins University. Their constructive comments were invaluable.

Finally, a huge helping of love and gratitude goes to my husband, Dr. Randolph Chase, and my children, Jordan Andrew and Rebecca Claire, for joining me on this adventure.

Notes

PROLOGUE

1. Personal communication, Bob Browning, U.S. Coast Guard historian, Washington, D.C., and Wayne Wheeler, president of the U.S. Lighthouse Society, San Francisco.
2. Gray Brechin, *Imperial San Francisco: Urban Power, Earthly Ruin* (Berkeley: University of California Press, 1999), pp. 126–127.
3. Ibid., pp. 274–279.
4. *More San Francisco Memoirs, 1852–1899: The Ripening Years,* ed. Malcolm E. Barker (San Francisco: Londonborn Publications, 1996), pp. 269 and 225–226. (The English novelist Anthony Trollope was unimpressed. "There is almost nothing in San Francisco that is worth seeing," he said. "There is an inferior menagerie of wild beasts, and a place called the Cliff house to which strangers are taken to hear seals bark." He added that the only noteworthy city feature was its stock exchange, which he pronounced even more "demoniac" than the one in Paris.)
5. Ibid., pp. 265–269.
6. Ibid., pp. 207–217.
7. For the flavor of immigrant life, see Marlon K. Hom, *Songs of Gold Mountain: Cantonese Rhymes from San Francisco Chinatown* (Berkeley: University of California Press, 1987).
8. Barker, ed., *More San Francisco Memoirs,* pp. 237–239.
9. George Rathmell, *Realms of Gold: The Colorful Writers of San Francisco, 1850–1950* (Berkeley: Creative Arts Book Co., 1998), pp. 174–176.

10. Philip P. Choy, Lorraine Dong, and Marlon K. Hom, *The Coming Man* (Seattle: University of Washington Press, 1995), p. 85.

11. Ibid., p. 92.

12. Joan B. Trauner, "The Chinese as Medical Scapegoats in San Francisco, 1870–1905," *California History* 57, no. 1 (Spring 1978): 70–87 (published by the California Historical Society).

13. "The hoodlum is a distinctive San Francisco product," wrote a writer for *Scribner's* named Samuel Williams. "One of his chief diversions when he is in a more pleasant mood and at peace with the world at large, is stoning Chinamen." Other etymologists trace the word to a mispronunciation of the Bavarian word *hodalump*, or the Irish *noodlum*, a corruption of the surname Muldoon. See Barker, ed., *More San Francisco Memoirs*, pp. 228–231.

14. Charles F. Adams, *The Magnificent Rogues of San Francisco* (Palo Alto: Pacific Books, 1998), p. 196.

15. "Wing Chung Knew the Game, But a 'Tin Roof' Came High," *San Francisco Examiner*, May 13, 1900.

16. Rathmell, *Realms of Gold*, pp. 77–78.

17. Harriet Lane Levy, *920 O'Farrell Street: A Jewish Girlhood in Old San Francisco* (Berkeley, Calif.: Heyday Books, 1996), pp.144–145.

18. Report of the Special Committee on the Condition of the Chinese Quarter, San Francisco Municipal Reports for the Fiscal Year 1884–1885, published by order of the San Francisco Board of Supervisors (San Francisco: W. M. Hinton & Co., 1885). Thanks to the Reverend Harry Chuck, Donaldina Cameron House, San Francisco, Calif., for sharing this document.

19. Bess Furman, *A Profile of the United States Public Health Service, 1798–1948* (Washington, D.C.: U.S. Department of Health, Education, and Welfare, 1973), pp. 230–231.

20. "Why San Francisco Is Plague-Proof," *San Francisco Examiner Sunday Magazine*, February 4, 1900.

21. Vernon B. Link, "A History of Plague in the United States," Public Health Monograph no. 26 (Washington, D.C.: U.S. Public Health Service, 1955).

22. Quarantine Officer Joseph Kinyoun thought the *Australia* was likely to have been the ship that introduced the plague that caused the March 1900 outbreak in San Francisco. See Joseph J. Kinyoun, Letter to Dr. Bailhache, August 9, 1900, p. 16, Joseph J. Kinyoun Manuscript Collection 1860–1913, Ms. C. 464, History of Medicine Division, National Library of Medicine, Bethesda, Md. For descriptions and photos of the *Australia*, thanks to the San Francisco Maritime National Historical Park Library.

The Year of the Rat

1. "Old Year Tooted Out, and the New One Noisily Welcomed," *San Francisco Chronicle,* January 1, 1900, p. 12.

2. Theodora Lau, *The Handbook of Chinese Horoscopes* (New York: Perennial Library, 1988), pp. 35–48.

3. Charles T. Gregg, *Plague: An Ancient Disease in the Twentieth Century* (Albuquerque: University of New Mexico Press, 1985), p. 171.

4. "The Story of Wong Chut King," *Chung Sai Yat Po,* March 8, 1900, translated by Prisca Hui. (Readers should note that the name of Wong Chut King varies in English-language newspaper accounts as Wing Chut King or Chick Gin, reflecting different pronunciations and transliterations. Regarding his village and district, Chinatown historian Him Mark Lai notes that speakers from Canton mingle their "n" and "l" sounds, so Ling Yup should be Ning Yup, short for Sunning district. The village of Pei Hang is a mingling of Cantonese and Mandarin. In this village, also known as Bak Hang, Wong was the dominant surname.)

5. Marlon K. Hom, *Songs of Gold Mountain: Cantonese Rhymes from San Francisco Chinatown* (Berkeley: University of California Press, 1987), pp. 308–322.

6. Descriptions of the pathology of plague and the progression of patients from infection to death, recounted by Gregg in *Plague,* pp. 113–128.

7. "The Story of Wong Chut King," *Chung Sai Yat Po,* March 8, 1900, p. 1. For explaining the significance of coffin shops and the meaning of *sau pan po,* or long-life boards, I am indebted to translator Prisca Hui. Historian Him Mark Lai adds his insight on cultural meanings of coffins and burial. *Sau pan* or *sau baan* means coffin, literally a longevity board. "Po" means store. He adds a better term might be *Cheung Sang Po,* which denotes a store for both long life and coffins.

8. "Quarantine of Chinatown," *Chung Sai Yat Po,* March 7, 1900, p. 1. Translated by Prisca Hui.

9. "Burning of Dead Body," *Chung Sai Yat Po,* March 21, 1900, p. 2. Translated by Prisca Hui.

10. "The Story of Wong Chut King," *Chung Sai Yat Po,* March 8, 1900, p. 1. Translated by Prisca Hui.

11. "No Results from Tests of Bacteriologist . . . Chinese Merchants Will Seek to Enjoin the Maintenance of Quarantine," *San Francisco Examiner,* March 9, 1900.

"A Lively Corpse"

1. Joseph J. Kinyoun, Letter to Dr. Bailhache, August 9, 1900, p. 41. Letters of Joseph J. Kinyoun, Ms. C. 464, History of Medicine Division, National Library of Medicine, Bethesda, Md.

2. Mrs. John Hendricks Kinyoun, Letter to "My Dear Husband," December 29, 1861, John Hendricks Kinyoun Papers, Genealogy Series, Rare Book, Manuscript, and Special Collections Library, Duke University.

3. John A. Garraty and Mark C. Carnes, *American National Biography*, vol. 12 (New York: Oxford University Press, 1999), p. 736.

4. John Hendricks Kinyoun Papers, Genealogy Series, Rare Book, Manuscript, and Special Collections Library, Duke University.

5. Garraty and Carnes, *American National Biography*, vol. 12, p. 736.

6. Bess Furman, *A Profile of the United States Public Health Service, 1798–1948* (Washington, D.C.: U.S. Department of Health, Education, and Welfare, 1973), p. 279.

7. Program, Complimentary Dinner to Joseph J. Kinyoun, Ms. C. 464, History of Medicine Division, National Library of Medicine, Bethesda, Md.

8. Joseph J. Kinyoun, Letter to "My Dear Aunt and Uncle," June 29, 1901, Joseph J. Kinyoun Manuscript Collection, Ms. C. 464, History of Medicine Division, National Library of Medicine, Bethesda, Md., pp. 1–2.

9. Joseph J. Kinyoun, Letter to Dr. Bailhache, Joseph J. Kinyoun Manuscript Collection, Ms. C. 464, History of Medicine Division, National Library of Medicine, Bethesda, Md., pp. 1–2.

10. Ibid., p. 27.

11. Ibid., p. 23.

12. Ibid., p. 50.

13. Ibid., pp. 1, 69.

14. Ibid., 50–51.

15. Ibid., pp. 16–17.

16. Joseph Kinyoun, Letter to Supervising Surgeon General, March 5, 1900, National Archives and Records Administration, Records Group 90, Central File 1897–1923, Box 627, Folder 5608, Folder January–May 1900, J. J. Kinyoun.

17. Kinyoun, Undated Telegram to Supervising Surgeon General, NARA, San Bruno, Calif., RG 90 (Public Health Service), Quarantine Station, Angel Island, Calif., Letters from the Surgeon General to the Medical Officer in Charge, July 1, 1891–July 1, 1918, Box 16, Vol. 3.

18. Charles T. Gregg, *Plague: An Ancient Disease in the Twentieth Century* (Albuquerque: University of New Mexico Press, 1985), pp. 40–41.

19. "Quarantine of Chinatown Raised, All Fears Proving Groundless," *San Francisco Examiner*, March 10, 1900.

THE BOY FROM CATFISH CREEK

1. Rupert Blue, Letter to Supervising Surgeon General, June 27, 1900, National Archives and Records Administration, Records Group 90, Central File 1897–1923, Box 616, Folder 3 of 3.
2. David T. Dennis, Kenneth L. Gage, et al., *Plague Manual: Epidemiology, Distribution, Surveillance and Control* (Geneva: World Health Organization, 1999), pp. 12–13.
3. Giovanni Boccaccio, *The Decameron,* translated by Guido Waldman (Oxford: Oxford University Press, 1998), pp. 12–13.
4. Daniel Defoe, *A Journal of the Plague Year* (London: Penguin Classics, 1986), pp. 27–28.
5. Philip Ziegler, *The Black Death* (Surrey, Eng.: Sutton Publishing Ltd., Bramley Books, Quadrillion Publishing Ltd., 1998), pp. 53–55.
6. Ibid., p. 37.
7. Major Arthur Henry Moorhead, "Plague in India," *The Military Surgeon,* March 1908, as cited in Frank Morton Todd, *Eradicating Plague from San Francisco* (San Francisco: C. Murdock and Co., 1909), p. 283.
8. W. W. Sellers, *A History of Marion County, South Carolina* (Columbia, S.C.: R. L. Bryan Co., 1902), p. 132.
9. Kate Lilly Blue, "Marion Men Lead Reconstruction," *News and Courier,* Charleston, S.C., March 11, 1934. South Caroliniana Library, University of South Carolina, Columbia, S.C.
10. Kate Lilly Blue, Historical Sketches of Marion County and Other Articles, SC R 975.757 Scrapbook Blu, Marion County, S.C., Public Library, South Carolina Room.
11. Personal communication of Miss Elizabeth McIntyre, one of Marion's venerable citizens, and Mr. Tommy Lett, curator of the Marion Museum, regarding the town's history and culture, during a reporting trip there in the summer of 2000.
12. Ibid.
13. Kate Lilly Blue, Letter to her cousin Theo, July 19, 1948. Blue Family Collection, South Caroliniana Library, University of South Carolina, Columbia, S.C.
14. Kate Lilly Blue, Letter to her cousin Mary, April 30, 1943. Blue Family Collection, South Caroliniana Library, University of South Carolina, Columbia, S.C.
15. Rupert Blue, Letter to Kate Lilly Blue, Latta, S.C., October 23, 1888. Collection of J. Michael Hughes.
16. Letters of John Gilchrist Blue, South Caroliniana Library, University of South Carolina, Columbia, S.C.
17. Details about the last illness and death of John Gilchrist Blue are drawn from at least four sources: Obituary of John Gilchrist Blue and

Letters of Victor Blue and John Gilchrist Blue, found in the Blue Family Collection, the South Caroliniana Library, University of South Carolina at Columbia. See also Letters of Rupert Blue to Kate Lilly Blue from collection of J. Michael Hughes, and W. W. Sellers, *A History of Marion County, South Carolina* (Columbia, S.C.: R. L. Bryan Co., 1902), p. 131.

18. Rupert Blue, Letter to Kate Lilly Blue, Albemarle Co., Va., October 27, 1889. Collection of J. Michael Hughes.

19. Rupert Blue, Letter to Kate Blue, Baltimore, Md., February 8, 1892. Collection of J. Michael Hughes.

20. Ibid., December 13, 1891. Collection of J. Michael Hughes.

21. Ibid., April 16, 1892. Collection of J. Michael Hughes.

22. Ibid., May 20, 1892. Collection of J. Michael Hughes.

23. Rupert Blue, Letter to Mrs. Annie M. Blue, December 16, 1910. Collection of J. Michael Hughes.

24. Reports of M. J. Rosenau and John Godfrey, Marine Hospital Service, Department of Health and Human Services, 1895–1896, Personnel Files of Rupert Blue, Division of Commissioned Personnel, Rockville, Md.

25. Letter of Rupert Blue to Kate Lilly Blue, Genoa, Italy, April 18, 1900. Collection of J. Michael Hughes.

26. Ibid., Norfolk, Va., January 24, 1906. Collection of J. Michael Hughes.

27. *Regulations Governing Uniforms of Officers and Employees of the United States Marine Hospital Service,* Treasury Department, Washington, D.C., Government Printing Office, 1893 and 1896 editions. Courtesy of U.S. Public Health Service Historian Dr. John Parascandola.

28. Thanks to U.S. Public Health Service historian John Parascandola for helpful discussions on the symbolism of the uniform.

29. This undated portrait of Rupert Blue in his Marine Hospital Service dress uniform, probably taken c. 1892 to 1895, is in the Blue Family collection at the South Caroliniana Library, University of South Carolina, Columbia, S.C.

Hiding the Dead

1. Henri H. Mollaret and Jacqueline Brossollet, *Alexandre Yersin, ou Le vainqueur de la peste* (Paris: Librairie Artheme Fayard, 1985), p. 137.

2. Ibid., p. 142.

3. Personal communication, Dr. Elisabeth Carniel, director, National Yersiniosis and World Health Organization Collaborating Center of the Pasteur Institute.

4. See Guenter B. Risse, " 'A Long Pull, a Strong Pull, and All Together':

San Francisco and Bubonic Plague, 1907–1908," *Bulletin of the History of Medicine* 66 (Spring 1992): 264. Most doctors regarded clinical examination of physical symptoms as a more reliable way to diagnose illness. "[T]he new bacteriology, with its microscope slides, germ cultures, and selective inoculations of experimental animals, remained an alien world for most of California's practitioners, trained in an earlier age."

5. "The Monkey Is Dead," *Chung Sai Yat Po,* March 14, 1900, p. 1.

6. Chinese Mortuary Records of the City and County of San Francisco, 1870–1933, National Archives and Records Administration, San Bruno, Calif., Cabinet 40, Drawer 9.

7. For another analysis of "yellow peril," Chinese and Japanese discrimination, and school segregation, see Gray Brechin, *Imperial San Francisco: Urban Power, Earthly Ruin* (Berkeley: University of California Press, 1999), pp. 156–168.

8. "Mayor Phelan Puts Himself on Record," *San Francisco Chronicle,* March 10, 1900.

9. Walter Wyman, Telegram to Surgeon Gassaway, March 8, 1900, NARA, San Bruno, Calif., Records Group 90, Quarantine Station, Angel Island, Calif., Series: Letters from Surgeon General to Medical Officer in Charge, July 1, 1891–July 1, 1918, Box 16, Folder, Volume 3.

10. Ibid.

11. J. A. Boyle, "How It Feels to Be Inoculated with Haffkine Serum," *San Francisco Examiner,* May 31, 1900, p. 3.

12. Mildred Crowl Martin, *Chinatown's Angry Angel: The Story of Donaldina Cameron* (Palo Alto, Calif.: Pacific Books, 1986), p. 78.

13. Ibid., pp. 58–61.

14. Ibid., pp. 77–78.

15. "Health Board Guarding the City Against the Plague," *San Francisco Examiner,* March 13, 1900.

16. "Suspiciously Small Chinatown Death Rate," *San Francisco Examiner,* March 18, 1900.

17. "Chinese Hide Their Sick from Officials," *San Francisco Examiner,* March 24, 1900. See also Guenter B. Risse, " 'A Long Pull, a Strong Pull, and All Together': San Francisco and Bubonic Plague, 1907–1908," *Bulletin of the History of Medicine* 66 (Spring 1992): 263.

18. W. G. Hay, M.D., "The Plague in Chinatown," *Occidental Medical Times,* August 1900, pp. 251–253.

19. "Suspiciously Small Chinatown Death Rate," *San Francisco Examiner,* March 18, 1900.

20. "In and Out of Kinyoun's Quarantine," *San Francisco Examiner,* March 16, 1900.

21. "Harassment Again," *Chung Sai Yat Po,* March 24, 1900, p. 1.

22. Brechin, *Imperial San Francisco*, pp. 178–179.
23. Guenter Risse, "The Politics of Fear: Bubonic Plague in San Francisco, California, 1900," *New Countries and Old Medicine* (Auckland, N.Z.: Pyramid Press, 1995), p. 9.
24. "City Plague Scare a Confessed Sham," *San Francisco Call*, March 27, 1900, p. 1.

A NEW QUARANTINE

1. Death of the sixteen-year-old cigar maker Lim Fa Muey from bubonic plague is recorded in the "Chinese Mortuary Record of the City and County of San Francisco, State of California," available on microfilm at the National Archives and Records Administration, Pacific Region, San Bruno, Calif. Dr. Kinyoun's recovery of plague bacteria from her glands is reported in an article ironically titled "Investigating Experts Inspect Chinatown and Fail to Find a Single Case of Any Illness," *San Francisco Call*, May 30, 1900, p. 1. Her symptoms listed here are those of classic bubonic plague as described by Charles T. Gregg, *Plague: An Ancient Disease in the Twentieth Century* (Albuquerque: University of New Mexico Press, 1985).
2. Affidavit of Minnie G. Worley, M.D., *Jew Ho* vs. *John Williamson et al.*, U.S. Circuit Court for the Ninth Circuit, Northern District of California, NARA, San Bruno, Calif., Records Group 21, Old Circuit Court, Northern District of California, Common Law Civil Cases, Box 746, Folder 12,940.
3. Ibid.
4. Walter Wyman, Letter to the Hon. Wu Ti-Fang, May 15, 1900, NARA, College Park, Md., Records Group 90, Central File 1897–1923, Box 636, 5608, Chinese Mortality 1897–1902, Folder 2 of 2. Although the government's official letter is addressed to the Chinese envoy as Wu Ti-Fang, San Francisco Chinatown historian Him Mark Lai points out that his name was Wu Ting-Fang.
5. Surgeon General Walter Wyman, Telegram to Quarantine Officer Kinyoun, May 15, 1900, *Wong Wai* vs. *Williamson*, Case File No. 12,937, Records Group 21, Old Circuit Court, Civil Cases, NARA, San Bruno, Calif. See also Charles J. McClain, *In Search of Equality: The Chinese Struggle Against Discrimination in Nineteenth-Century America* (Berkeley: University of California Press, 1994), p. 244.
6. Surgeon General Wyman, Telegram to Kinyoun, February 10, 1900: "Evidence has accumulated showing rats are chief means of conveying plague from port to port." NARA, San Bruno, Calif., Records

Group 90, Quarantine Station, Angel Island, Letters from Surgeon General to the Medical Officer in Charge, July 1, 1891 to July 1, 1918, Box 16, Vol. 3. The *San Francisco Examiner,* on May 18, 1900, published a story headlined FLEAS ARE CARRIERS OF THE PLAGUE; BACILLI FOUND IN INSECTS' STOMACHS BY AUSTRALIAN DOCTORS. Apparently, nobody linked the clues.

7. Kinyoun, Letter to Dr. Bailhache, August 9, 1900, from the Joseph J. Kinyoun Manuscript Collection 464, History of Medicine Division, National Library of Medicine, Bethesda, Md., p. 5.

8. Thanks to Chinatown historian Him Mark Lai for his helpful interpretation of "wolf doctor."

9. "The Reason for Immunization," *Chung Sai Yat Po,* May 19, 1900, p. 1.

10. Mildred Crowl Martin recounts this scene in *Chinatown's Angry Angel: The Story of Donaldina Cameron* (Palo Alto, Calif.: Pacific Books, 1986), p. 78, noting that the missionary attributed the fear of the shot to ignorance rather than well-taken objections to vaccine dangers.

11. "The Reason for Immunization," *Chung Sai Yat Po,* May 19, 1900, p. 1.

12. "Interstate Quarantine Regulations to Prevent the Spread of Plague in the United States," May 22, 1900, NARA, Records Group 90, Central File 1897–1923, Box 636, File 5608, Chinese Mortality 1897–1902, File 2 of 2. See also Guenter B. Risse, " 'A Long Pull, a Strong Pull, and All Together': San Francisco and Bubonic Plague, 1907–1908," *Bulletin of the History of Medicine* 66 (Spring 1992): 265. See also *Wong Wai* vs. *John M. Williamson et al.,* NARA, San Bruno, Calif., Records Group 21, No. 12,937.

13. *Wong Wai* vs. *John M. Williamson et al.,* in the United States Circuit Court, Ninth Circuit, Northern District of California, NARA, San Bruno, Calif., Records Group 21, No. 12,937.

14. McClain, *In Search of Equality,* p. 254.

15. Opinion in *Wong Wai* vs. *John M. Williamson et al.,* NARA, San Bruno, Calif., Records Group 21, No. 12,937.

16. "Board of Health Confesses to a Famous Expert That There Is No Bubonic Plague in This City," *San Francisco Call,* May 29, 1900, p. 2.

17. "Cordon of City Police Is Drawn Around Chinatown," *San Francisco Examiner,* May 30, 1900, p. 3.

18. Joseph Kinyoun, Letter to Dr. Bailhache, National Library of Medicine, p. 36.

19. "Investigating Experts Inspect Chinatown and Fail to Find a Single Case of Any Illness," *San Francisco Call,* May 30, 1900, p. 1.

20. Letter to Dr. Bailhache, Kinyoun Letters, National Library of Medicine, pp. 37–38.

21. "Sporadic Case of Bubonic Plague Discovered, but There Is Absolutely No Need for Alarm," *San Francisco Call*, May 31, 1900, p. 1.

22. "Autopsy of Dang Hong," *Chung Sai Yat Po*, May 30, 1900, p. 2.

23. "Danger of Plague Has Passed and Vigilance Will Ensure Complete Safety to the City," *San Francisco Call*, June 1, 1900, p. 2.

24. "Dr. Shrady Dined by Mayor Phelan," *San Francisco Call*, June 3, 1900.

25. Joseph J. Kinyoun, Letter to "My Dear Aunt and Uncle," June 29, 1901. From the Joseph J. Kinyoun, Manuscript Collection 464, History of Medicine Division, National Library of Medicine, p. 8¾.

26. "San Francisco Free from Danger of Contagion," *San Francisco Call*, June 2, 1900, p. 1.

27. Letter to Dr. Bailhache, Kinyoun Letters, National Library of Medicine, p. 38.

THE WOLF DOCTOR

1. "Health Board Vents Animus on Pillsbury," *San Francisco Call*, June 3, 1900.

2. *Jew Ho* vs. *John M. Williamson et al.*, National Archives and Records Administration, San Bruno, Calif., Records Group 21, U.S. District Court, Old Circuit Court, Northern District of California, Common Law Civil Cases, Box 746, Folder 12,940.

3. "Signs of Riot Among the Chinese in Quarantine," *San Francisco Call*, June 8, 1900.

4. "Officials Investigating the Chinese Blackmail Scandal," *San Francisco Call*, June 10, 1900, p. 1.

5. Ibid.

6. "Riot Raised Among Quarantined Chinese," *San Francisco Call*, June 12, 1900.

7. "Another Hearing of Lawsuit," *Chung Sai Yat Po*, June 14, 1900.

8. "De Haven Strikes First Blow at the Quarantine," *San Francisco Call*, June 13, 1900.

9. "No Plague Says Governor Gage," *San Francisco Call*, June 14, 1900. See also Guenter B. Risse, " 'A Long Pull, a Strong Pull, and All Together': San Francisco and Bubonic Plague, 1907–1908," *Bulletin of the History of Medicine* 66 (Spring 1992): 266.

10. *Jew Ho* vs. *John M. Williamson et al.*

11. Ibid.

12. "Chinatown Quarantine Raised by Order of Federal Court," *San Francisco Examiner*, June 16, 1900. For a legal analysis of the importance of the quarantine, *Wong Wai*, and *Jew Ho* cases, see also

Charles McClain, *In Search of Equality: The Chinese Struggle Against Discrimination in Nineteenth-Century America* (Berkeley: University of California Press, 1994), pp. 234–276.

13. J. J. Kinyoun, Telegram to Pacific Coast Steamship Company, June 15, 1900, cited in *Wong Wai* vs. *John M. Williamson et al.*, NARA, Records Group 21, U.S. District Court, Old Circuit Court, Northern District of California, Common Law Civil Cases, Box 746, Folder 12,937.

14. J. J. Kinyoun, Telegram to Surgeon General Wyman, June 16, 1900, NARA, Records Group 90, Box 627, Folder June 1900, J. J. Kinyoun.

15. J. J. Kinyoun, Telegram to State Board of Health of Louisiana, June 15, 1900, as cited in *Wong Wai* vs. *John M Williamson et al.*, NARA, San Bruno, Calif., Records Group 21, U.S. District Court, Old Circuit Court, Northern District of California, Common Law Civil Cases, Box 746, Folder 12,937.

16. Republican State Central Committee of California, Telegram to President McKinley, qtd. in "California Is Subjected to an Unparalleled Outrage," *San Francisco Call*, June 17, 1900, p. 23.

17. "Kinyoun Begs for Mercy in Court," *San Francisco Call*, June 18, 1900, p. 10.

18. "President McKinley Answers Appeal of State and Raises Kinyoun Quarantine," *San Francisco Call*, June 19, 2000, p. 5.

19. Joseph J. Kinyoun, Letter to Dr. Bailhache, August 9, 1900, Joseph J. Kinyoun Manuscript Collection, Ms. 464, in History of Medicine Collection, National Library of Medicine, Bethesda, Md., p. 9.

20. Excerpts of testimony are from Transcript of Kinyoun's Contempt Hearing in *Wong Wai* vs. *John M. Williamson et al.*, June 25–July 2, 1900, NARA, San Bruno, Calif., Records Group 21, U.S. District Court, Old Circuit Court, Northern District of California, Common Law Civil Cases, Box 746, Folder 12,937.

21. Rupert Blue, Letter to the Supervising Surgeon General, June 27, 1900, NARA, Records Group 90, Central File 1897–1923, Box 616, File 3 of 3.

22. The children's dinner discussion is recounted in Kinyoun's Letter to Dr. Bailhache, Kinyoun Ms. C. 464, History of Medicine Division, National Library of Medicine, Bethesda, Md., p. 17.

23. "Kinyoun Purged of Contempt by Circuit Court," *San Francisco Call*, July 4, 1900.

24. The conference on the ferry boat is also recounted in Kinyoun's Letter to Dr. Bailhache, Kinyoun Ms. C. 464, History of Medicine Division, National Library of Medicine, Bethesda, Md., p. 11.

25. "Oust the Fakers," *San Francisco Call*, June 26, 1900, p. 6.

WHITE MEN'S FUNERALS

1. Details of William Murphy's case come from several sources: His alleged opium addiction was reported in the *Sacramento Bee,* January 12, 1901, p. 1. His diagnosis with plague at autopsy comes from Kinyoun's letter to Dr. Bailhache, Joseph J. Kinyoun Manuscript Collection, Ms. C. 464, History of Medicine Division, National Library of Medicine, Bethesda, Md., p. 14.

2. J. J. Kinyoun, Letter to Dr. Bailhache, Joseph J. Kinyoun Manuscript Collection, Ms. C. 464, History of Medicine Division, National Library of Medicine, Bethesda, Md., p. 14.

3. Ibid., pp. 53–55.

4. Ibid., p. 53.

5. Ibid., p. 20.

6. James Moloney, surgeon of the SS *Coptic,* Letter to the Surgeon in Charge, U.S. Marine Hospital Service, San Francisco, September 30, 1900, National Archives and Records Administration, Records Group 90, Box 627, Folder June 1900, J. J. Kinyoun.

7. Ibid.

8. Ibid.

9. J. J. Kinyoun, Letter to the Surgeon General, October 10, 1900, NARA, College Park, Md., Records Group 90, Box 627, Folder June 1900, J. J. Kinyoun.

10. J. J. Kinyoun, Letter to Dr. Bailhache, pp. 18–19.

11. J. J. Kinyoun, Letter to Surgeon General, December 29, 1900, NARA, College Park, Md., Records Group 90, Box 627, Folder June 1900, J. J. Kinyoun.

12. "Dr. Kinyoun May Move His Drugs to Other Parts," *San Francisco Call,* December 20, 1900.

13. "Dr. Kinyoun May Soon Be Transferred," *San Francisco Call,* December 22, 1900.

14. Wong Chung, Letter to Dr. Kinyoun, December 18, 1900, and the complaint of *Wong Chung* vs. *J. J. Kinyoun et al.,* both found in NARA, College Park, Md., Records Group 90, Box 627, Folder 5608, 1901, J. J. Kinyoun.

15. J. J. Kinyoun, Letter to the Surgeon General of December 6, 1900, as cited in Letter to Dr. Bailhache, p. 75.

16. "Commercial Outlook," *San Francisco Call,* December 31, 1900, p. 6.

17. Kinyoun, Letter to Dr. Bailhache, p. 68.

18. "The Doom of Kinyoun," *San Francisco Chronicle,* December 28, 1900, editorial page (from NARA, College Park, Md., Records Group 90, Box 627, Folder June 1900, J. J. Kinyoun).

19. Kinyoun, Letter to Dr. Bailhache, p. 68.

20. "Plague Is the Burden of the Governor's Message," *Sacramento Bee*, January 9, 1901, pp. 2–4. Emphasis added.

21. Ibid.

22. "State Senate Demands Dr. Kinyoun's Removal," *San Francisco Call*, January 24, 1901.

23. Joseph J. Kinyoun, Letter to "My Dear Aunt and Uncle," June 29, 1901. From the Joseph J. Kinyoun Manuscript Collection, Ms. C. 464, in the History of Medicine Division, National Library of Medicine, Bethesda, Md., p. 25.

24. J. J. Kinyoun, Telegram to Supervising Surgeon General, January 10, 1901, NARA, College Park, Md., Records Group 90, Box 627, Folder 5608, 1901, J. J. Kinyoun.

25. Joseph J. Kinyoun, Letter to "My Dear Aunt and Uncle," Detroit, Mich., June 29, 1901, National Library of Medicine, p. 26.

26. "Scathing Arraignment by Dr. Williamson," *Sacramento Bee*, January 16, 1901, p. 4.

27. Lewellys F. Barker, *Time and the Physician* (New York: G. P. Putnam's Sons, 1942), pp. 82–83.

28. J. H. White attributes the eviction from the lab to the university president, in Telegram to Surgeon General Wyman, February 4, 1901, NARA, Records Group 90, Box 625, Folder 5608, File 3 of 4. Kinyoun cites the threat of lost funding for the action in his letter to "My Dear Aunt and Uncle," p. 28. Kinyoun Manuscript Collection, Ms. C. 464, History of Medicine Division, National Library of Medicine, p. 28.

29. Special Commission on Plague, Letter to Surgeon General Wyman, NARA, College Park, Md. Records Group 90, Central File 1897–1923, Box 637, Folder 1899–1909, Surgeon General.

30. "Federal Plague Commission Has Practically Finished," *Sacramento Bee*, February 18, 1901, p. 1.

31. "Gage in the Dumps over That 'Conference,' " *Sacramento Bee*, February 19, 1901, p. 2, col. 4.

32. "More Pressure upon M'Kinley," *Sacramento Bee*, February 28, 1901, p. 1.

33. Joseph Kinyoun, Telegram to Surgeon General, March 1, 1901, NARA, College Park, Md., Records Group 90, Central File 1897–1923, Box 627, Folder 5608, File 1901, J. J. Kinyoun.

34. J. H. White, Letter to "Dear Dr.," February 26, 1901, NARA, Records Group 90, Central File 1897–1923, Box 625, Folder 5608, File 3 of 4.

35. Ibid., March 7, 1901, NARA, Records Group 90, Box 625, Folder 5608, File 3 of 4.

SEAL OF SILENCE

1. Telegram of Geo. C. Perkins and Thos. R. Bard, Febuary 20, 1901, for information of Gen. O. L. Spaulding, Assistant Treasury Secretary, National Archives and Records Administration, College Park, Md., Records Group 90, Central File 1897–1923, Box 636, Folder 5608, Chinese Mortality 1897–1902, Conference '02–'03, Memoranda '01–'03, Autopsies '02–'03.

2. Geo. C. Perkins, Letter to Hon O. L. Spaulding, Assistant Treasury Secretary, February 21, 1901, NARA, College Park, Md., Records Group 90, Central File 1897–1923, Box 636, Folder 5608, Chinese Mortality 1897–1902, Conference '02–'03, Memoranda '01–'03, Autopsies '02–'03.

3. Walter Wyman, Personal and Confidential Letter to Doctor Victor Vaughan, February 20, 1901, NARA, Records Group 90, Central File 1897–1923, Box 636, Folder 5608, Chinese Mortality 1897–1902, File 2 of 2. Wyman wrote:

   > Dear Doctor Vaughan,
   > I telegraphed you today, asking you to use your efforts to prevent publication of any information that might reach Ann Arbor concerning work of Commission in San Francisco, out of superabundant caution, having no reason to suppose at all that the seal of silence will be broken by any of the commission. Yet inferences might be drawn from their work and I know that the Associated Press in Ann Arbor is very active. The object of silence is for the purpose of bringing the Governor around to work with us, which will be more difficult if the matter is made public. With regards, Sincerely Yours, WALTER WYMAN, Surgeon-General, Marine Hospital Service.

4. "Bubonic Plague Exists in San Francisco and Probably in Other Cities on the Coast," *Sacramento Bee*, March 6, 1901, p. 1.

5. "Infamous Compact Signed by Wyman," *Sacramento Bee*, March 16, 1901, p. 1, col. 3.

6. "Bubonic Plague 'News' Comes from Washington," *Sacramento Bee*, March 11, 1901, p. 8, col. 4.

7. J. J. Kinyoun, Telegram to Supervising Surgeon General, March 9, 1901, NARA, College Park, Md., Records Group 90, Central File 1897–1923, Box 627, Folder 5608, 1901, J. J. Kinyoun.

8. Walter Wyman, Telegram to Surgeon Kinyoun, March 11, 1901, NARA, San Bruno, Calif., Records Group 90, Subgroup Quarantine Station, Angel Island, Calif. Series Letters from the Surgeon General to the Medical Officer in Charge, Accession, July 1, 1891, to July 1, 1918, Box 16, Vol. 4.

9. J. H. White, Letter to "Dear Doctor," March 7, 1901, NARA, College Park, Md., Records Group 90, Central File 1897–1923, Box 625, Folder 5608, File 3 of 4.

10. Ibid., March 19, 1901, NARA, College Park, Md., Records Group 90, Central File 1897–1923, Box, 625, Folder 5608, File 3 of 4.

11. Letter of Lewellys F. Barker to "My Dear Dr. Wyman," April 6, 1901, NARA, College Park, Md., Records Group 90, Central File 1897–1923, Box 637, Folder 1899–1909, Surgeon General.

12. Letter of Lewellys F. Barker, to "My Dear Dr. Wyman," April 11, 1901, NARA, College Park, Md., Records Group 90, Central File 1897–1923, Box 637, Folder 1899–1909, Surgeon General.

13. Lewellys F. Barker, *Time and the Physician* (New York: G. P. Putman's Sons, 1942), p. 114.

14. F. G. Novy, Telegram to Surgeon General Wyman, April 5, 1901, NARA, College Park, Md., Records Group 90, Central File 1897–1923, Box 637, Folder 5608, 1899–1909, Surgeon General. See also F. G. Novy, Letter to Surgeon General Wyman, with attached case report written for *Journal of the American Medical Association*, April 9, 1901, NARA, College Park, Md., Records Group 90, Central File 1897–1923, Box 637, Folder 1899–1909, Surgeon General. See also Howard Markel, "Prescribing 'Arrowsmith,' " *New York Times*, September 24, 2000, for impact of the Hare case on Sinclair Lewis's novel.

15. Charles T. Gregg, *Plague: An Ancient Disease in the Twentieth Century* (Albuquerque: University of New Mexico Press, 1985), pp. 90–91.

16. Walter Wyman, Letter to J. J. Kinyoun, April 6, 1901, NARA, San Bruno, Calif., Records Group 90, Central File 1897–1923, Subgroup Quarantine Station, Angel Island, Calif., Series: Letters from the Surgeon General to the Medical Officer in Charge, July 1, 1891–July 1, 1918, Box 16, Vol. 4.

17. J. J. Kinyoun, Letter to "My Dear Aunt and Uncle," from the Joseph J. Kinyoun (1860–1913) Manuscript Collection, Ms. C. 464, in the History of Medicine Division, National Library of Medicine, Bethesda, Md., pp. 32, 34.

18. "Truth Suppression and Not Plague Suppression," *Sacramento Bee,* April 22, 1901, p. 4, col. 3.

19. "Kinyoun Says He Is Falsely Accused," *Sacramento Bee*, May 6, 1901, p. 5, col. 6.

20. J. J. Kinyoun, Letter to "My Dear Aunt and Uncle," June 29, 1901, from the J. J. Kinyoun papers, Ms. C. 464, in the History of Medicine Division, National Library of Medicine, Bethesda, Md, p. 40. For an analysis of Kinyoun's downfall, see also Guenter B. Risse, " 'A Long Pull, a Strong Pull, and All Together': San Francisco and Bubonic Plague, 1907–1908," *Bulletin of the History of Medicine* 66 (Spring

1992): "Kinyoun . . . became the target of a systematic campaign of vituperation and was denounced as an enemy of San Francisco."

21. J. J. Kinyoun, Letter to "Dear Doctor Bailhache," August 9, 1900, Joseph J. Kinyoun, Ms. C. 464, History of Medicine Collection, National Library of Medicine, Bethesda, Md., p. 61.

New Blood

1. J. H. White, Letter to "Dear Doctor," April 18, 1901, National Archives and Records Administration, College Park, Md., Records Group 90, Central File 1897–1923, Box 625, Folder 5608, File 3 of 4.

2. "Colorado's Quarantine Still Maintained," *Sacramento Bee,* March 28, 1901.

3. "Plague Report at Last Sees the Light of Day," *Sacramento Bee,* April 15, 1901. White protests that he wasn't the source of the leak in his "Dear Doctor" letter cited above. Dr. Barker wrote Surgeon General Wyman asking for copies of the official report in a letter of April 27, 1901, located at NARA, College Park, Md., Records Group 90, Central File 1897–1923, Box 637, Folder 1899–1909, Surgeon General.

4. M. J. White, Letter to Surgeon J. H. White, April 23, 1901, NARA, College Park, Md., Records Group 90, Central File 1897–1923, Box 625, Folder 5608, File 3 of 4.

5. J. H. White, Letter to Dr. Wyman, April 24, 1901, NARA, College Park, Md., Records Group 90, Central File 1897–1923, Box 625, Folder 5608, File 2 of 4.

6. J. H. White, Personal Letter to Surgeon General Walter Wyman, April 30, 1901, NARA, College Park, Md., Records Group 90, Central File 1897–1923, Box 625, Folder 5608, 2 of 4.

7. J. H. White, Letter to "Dear Doctor," May 10, 1901, NARA, College Park, Md., Records Group 90, Central File 1897–1923, Box 625, Folder 5608, File 2 of 4.

8. J. H. White, Telegram to Wyman, May 4, 1901, NARA, College Park, Md., Records Group 90, Central File 1897–1923, Box 625, Folder 5608, File 3 of 4.

9. J. H. White, Letter to "Dear Doctor," May 10, 1901, NARA, College Park, Md., Records Group 90, Central File 1897–1923, Box 625, Folder 5608, File 2 of 4.

10. J. H. White, Letter to "His Excellency Henry T. Gage, Governor of the State of California," May 18, 1901, NARA, College Park, Md., Records Group 90, Central File 1897–1923, Box 624, Folder 2 of 2.

11. J. H. White, Letter to Supervising Surgeon General, May 29, 1901, NARA, College Park, Md., Records Group 90, Central File (1897–1923), Box 624, File 2 of 2.

12. Ibid.

13. J. H. White, Personal Letter to Surgeon General Walter Wyman, April 30, 1901, NARA, College Park, Md., Records Group 90, Central File 1897–1923, Box 625, Folder 5608, File 2 of 4.

14. "McKinley Reaches City, Not as President, but as Devoted Husband, Solicitous for the Welfare of His Beloved Wife," *San Francisco Call*, May 13, 1901.

15. Details of the McKinleys' visit to San Francisco made headlines for two weeks, including these details from the *San Francisco Call*, May 13–26, 1901.

16. Rupert Blue, Letter to Supervising Surgeon General, July 2, 1901, NARA, College Park, Md., Records Group 90, Central File 1897–1923, Box 616, File 3 of 3.

17. Walter Wyman, Letter to Henry T. Gage, July 5, 1901, NARA, College Park, Md., Records Group 90, Central File 1897–1923, Box 624, File 2 of 2.

18. H. Ryfkogel, Letter to Drs. Regensburger, Carpenter, Evans, Dodge, and Kurozawa, July 8, 1901, NARA, College Park, Md., Records Group 90, Central File 1897–1923, Box 627, Folder 5608, 1901, J. J. Kinyoun.

19. Autopsy Number 63: Miyo, NARA, College Park, Md., Records Group 90, Central File 1897–1923, Box 625, Folder 5608, File 2 of 4.

20. Autopsy Number 64: Shina, NARA, College Park, Md., Records Group 90, Central File 1897–1923, Box 625, Folder 5608, File 2 of 4.

21. Rupert Blue, Telegram to Surgeon General Wyman, July 10, 1901, NARA, College Park, Md., Records Group 90, Central File 1897–1923, Box 616, File 3 of 3.

22. "Deaths of Two Prostitutes in Chinatown Suspected of Having Plague," *Chung Sai Yat Po*, July 12, 1901.

23. Rupert Blue, Letter to Surgeon General, July 20, 1901, NARA, College Park, Md., Records Group 90, Central File 1897–1923, Box 616, File 3 of 3.

24. Rupert Blue, Personal Letter to Surgeon General Wyman, July 11, 1901, NARA, College Park, Md., Records Group 90, Central File 1897–1923, Box 616, File 3 of 3.

25. Rupert Blue, Letter to Surgeon General Walter Wyman, July 25, 1901, NARA, College Park, Md., Records Group 90, Box 616, File 3 of 3.

26. "Striking Teamsters Go on the Warpath," *San Francisco Call*, August 29, 1901, p. 1.

27. M. J. White, Letter to Surgeon General, September 3, 1901, NARA, College Park, Md., Records Group 90, Central File 1897–1923, Box 625, File 2 of 4.

28. "State Will Pay Coin for 'Shadowing' Work," *San Francisco Call*, Sep-

tember 6, 1901, and "What Ryfkogel Thinks of Gage," *San Francisco Call,* September 7, 1901. These one-hundred-year-old clippings on the case were attached to federal public health service plague files with a handwritten note in the margin: "Wouldn't this jar you?" NARA, College Park, Md., Records Group 90, Central File 1897–1923, Box 616, File 3 of 3.

THE BITE OF A FLEA

1. Rupert Blue, Personal Letter to General Walter Wyman, September 25, 1901, National Archives and Records Administration, Records Group 90, Central File 1897–1923, Box 616, File 3 of 3.
2. Marlon K. Hom, *Songs of Gold Mountain: Cantonese Rhymes from San Francisco Chinatown* (Berkeley: University of California Press, 1987), p. 29.
3. M. J. White, Letter to the Surgeon General, September 14, 1901, NARA, Records Group 90, Central File 1897–1923, Box 625, Folder 5608, File 2 of 4.
4. Rupert Blue, Letter to the Surgeon General, September 23, 1901, NARA, Records Group 90, Central File 1897–1923, Box 616, File 3 of 3.
5. Rupert Blue, Personal Letter to Surgeon General Walter Wyman, September 25, 1901, NARA, Records Group 90, Central File 1897–1923, Box 616, File 3 of 3.
6. Rupert Blue, Letter to Supervising Surgeon General, October 4, 1901, NARA, Records Group 90, Central File 1897–1923, Box 616, File 3 of 3.
7. Henri H. Mollaret and Jacqueline Brossolet, *Alexandre Yersin, ou Le vainqueur de la peste* (Paris: Librairie Artheme Fayard, 1985), p. 165.
8. *The Bubonic Plague,* a monograph by Walter Wyman, surgeon general, Marine Hospital Service (Washington, D.C.: Government Printing Office, 1900), pp. 25–26.

WONG CHUNG, DETECTIVE

1. Rupert Blue, Personal Letter to Surgeon General Wyman, September 29, 1901, National Archives and Records Administration, Records Group 90, Central File 1897–1923, Box 616, File 3 of 3.
2. M. J. White, Letter to Passed Assistant Surgeon Rupert Blue, September 27, 1901, NARA, Records Group 90, Central File 1897–1923, Box 616, File 3 of 3.
3. Rupert Blue, Personal Letter to Walter Wyman, October 18, 1901,

NARA, College Park, Md., Records Group 90, Central File 1897–1923, Box 616, File 3 of 3.

4. The birth of the Ruef-Schmitz alliance is recounted by Walton Bean in *Boss Ruef's San Francisco* (Berkeley: University of California Press, 1952), pp. 20–21. It is also treated by Charles F. Adams in *The Magnificent Rogues of San Francisco* (Palo Alto: Pacific Books, 1998), pp. 222–246.

5. "Crowds Cheer for Schmitz," *San Francisco Chronicle*, November 6, 1901, p. 2.

6. Bean, *Boss Ruef's San Francisco*, p. 29.

7. Mark White, Letters to the Supervising Surgeon General, on December 23, 1901, and December 30, 1901, and Telegram of January 13, 1902, NARA, Records Group 90, Central File 1897–1923, Box 625, Folders 5608, 5624, and 5608.

8. "Big House to See Sponge Thrown Up; Once More San Francisco Pays Dear for Witnessing an Easy Money Game," *San Francisco Chronicle*, sports page, November 16, 1901.

9. Bess Furman, *A Profile of the United States Public Health Service, 1798–1948* (Washington, D.C.: U.S. Department of Health, Education, and Welfare, 1973). The late Bess Furman interviewed Surgeon General Blue's secretary and contemporaries. Her cryptic handwritten notes on this exchange are filed at the National Library of Medicine, in Bethesda, Md. (Ms. C. 202, HMD Manuscripts, NLM012683199, Furman, Bess, 1894–1969, project materials pertaining to a history of the U.S. Public Health Service, Box 16, Chapters 12–13, steno pad).

10. "Chinese Go East to Lecture and Sing Against Exclusion," *San Francisco Examiner*, December 5, 1901, p. 6, col. 1.

11. "Exclude Chinese, Build Up the Navy—Roosevelt," *San Francisco Examiner*, December 4, 1901, p. 3, col. 1.

12. "Some Scientific Prophecies," *San Francisco Examiner*, New Year's Supplement, January 1, 1902, p. 3, col. 1.

13. M. J. White, Letter to the Surgeon General, April 22, 1902, NARA, College Park, Md., Records Group 90, Central File 1897–1923, Box 624, File 1 of 2.

14. "Mayor Schmitz Removes Four Members of Board of Health," *San Francisco Examiner*, March 26, 1902, p. 1.

15. Affidavit of Wong Chung, May 19, 1902, and M. J. White, Letters to Supervising Surgeon General, May 20 and 21, 1901, NARA, College Park, Md., Records Group 90, Central File 1897–1923, Box 624, File 2 of 2.

16. M. J. White, Letter to the Surgeon General, May 22, 1902, NARA, Records Group 90, Central File 1897–1923, Box 624, Folder 5608, File 1 of 2.

17. H. Brett Melendy and Benjamin F. Gilbert, *The Governors of California* (Georgetown, Calif.: Talisman Press, 1965), pp. 270–274.

18. M. J. White, Letter to Surgeon General, May 30, 1902, NARA, Records Group 90, Central File 1897–1923, Box 624, File 2 of 2.

19. M. J. White details the deaths of the seventeen-year-old boy and the cook Huie Chong Bow in two letters to the surgeon general, both dated September 24, 1902, NARA, College Park, Md., Records Group 90, Central File 1897–1923, Box 624, File 1 of 2.

20. M. J. White, Telegram to Surgeon General Wyman, October 7, 1902, NARA, College Park, Md., Records Group 90, Central File 1897–1923, Box 624, File 2 of 2.

21. M. J. White, Letter to the Surgeon General, October 8, 1902, NARA, Records Group 90, Central File 1897–1923, Box 624, File 2 of 2.

22. John Hay, Letter to the Secretary of the Treasury, October 11, 1902, NARA, Records Group 90, Central File 1897–1923, Box 624, File 2 of 2.

"Send Blue ASAP"

1. Resolutions of the State and Provincial Boards of Health of North America at the Annual Meeting held at New Haven, October 28–29, 1902, National Archives and Records Administration, Records Group 90, Central File 1897–1923, Box 636, Folder 5608, File 1 of 2.

2. M. J. White, Letter to Surgeon General, October 29, 1902, NARA, Records Group 90, Box 624, File 2 of 2. Caswell's death and his intemperate habits are noted in "List of Cases of Plague" in San Francisco, Calif., from March 6, 1900, to December 11, 1902, filed at NARA, Records Group 90, Central File 1897–1923, Box 616, File 2 of 2.

3. A. H. Glennan, Letter to the Surgeon General, October 21, 1902, NARA, Records Group 90, Central File 1897–1923, Box 626, Folder 5608, 1902, Surgeon Glennan. Glennan recaps his audience with the governor in this letter, expressing shock at the governor's crude eruptions, and bowdlerized his outburst as "That ____-____ plague again."

4. M. J. White, Letter to the Surgeon General, September 12, 1902, NARA, Records Group 90, Central File 1897–1923, Box 624, File 1 of 2.

5. The account of this meeting is from M. J. White's Letter to the Surgeon General of November 4, 1902, NARA, Records Group 90, Central File 1897–1923, Box 624, File 2 of 2.

6. "Plague Fake Is Exposed; Dr. Glennan Says Bubonic Tales Are False," *San Francisco Call*, December 12, 1902, p. 1 col. 1.

7. Bess Furman, *A Profile of the United States Public Health Service*,

1798–1948 (Washington, D.C.: U.S. Department of Health, Education, and Welfare, 1973), pp. 251–252.

8. Walter Wyman, Letter to Edmond Souchon, January 11, 1903, NARA, Records Group 90, Central File 1897–1923, Box 636, Folder 5608, File 1 of 2.

9. A. H. Glennan, "Dear General" Letter to Wyman, January 14, 1903, NARA, Records Group 90, Central File 1897–1923, Box 616, File 1 of 3.

10. "The Plague Conference Held at Washington, D.C., January 19, 1903," *American Medicine*, January 31, 1903, NARA, Records Group 90, Central File 1897–1923, Box 624, File 1 of 2.

11. Walter Wyman, Telegram to A. H. Glennan, January 28, 1903, NARA, Records Group 90, Central File 1897–1923, Box 636, Folder 5608, Chinese Mortality, '97–'02, File 2 of 2.

12. A. H. Glennan, Telegram to Surgeon General Wyman, January 29, 1903, NARA, Records Group 90, Central File 1897–1923, Box 636, Folder 5608, Chinese Mortality, '97–'02, File 2 of 2.

THE PERIMETER WIDENS

1. Rupert Blue, Letter to Miss Kate Blue, January 31, 1903, Collection of J. Michael Hughes.

2. A. H. Glennan, Letter to the Surgeon General, February 12, 1903, National Archives and Records Administration, Records Group 90, Central File 1897–1923, Box 626, Folder 5608, 1903, Glennan.

3. Rupert Blue, entry of February 15, 1903, in the *Plague Journal 1901–1905*, of Drs. Currie, Blue, et al., National Library of Medicine.

4. "Chinese Complain of Unsanitary Conditions," *San Francisco Examiner*, April 5, 1903, p. 28, col. 7, and "Legal Obstruction to Chinatown Cleaning," *San Francisco Examiner*, April 7, 1903, p. 6, col. 2.

5. Rupert Blue, Letter to the Surgeon General, July 23, 1903, NARA, Records Group 90, Central File 1897–1923, Box 616, File 1 of 2.

6. Rupert Blue to Walter Wyman, August 17, 1903, NARA, Records Group 90, Central File 1897–1923, Box 616, File 1 of 3.

7. "Only Chinatown's Removal Will Bring the City Security," *Merchant's Association Review*, August 1903, p. 2, NARA, Records Group 90, Central File 1897–1923, Box 646, File 4 of 6.

8. Rupert Blue, Letter to Kate Lilly Blue, San Francisco, September 23, 1903. Collection of J. Michael Hughes.

9. Walton Bean, *Boss Ruef's San Francisco* (Berkeley: University of California Press, 1952), p. 41.

10. Rupert Blue, Letter to Walter Wyman, December 9, 1903, NARA, Records Group 90, Central File 1897–1923, Box 616, File 1 of 2.

11. "Says City Is Seat of Satan," *San Francisco Chronicle,* May 24, 1904.
12. *Sacramento Bee,* March 1, 1904, p. 1.
13. Rupert Blue, Personal Letter to Surgeon General Wyman, January 15, 1904, NARA, Records Group 90, Central File 1897–1923, Box 617, File 1 of 2.

The Seamstresses

1. Telegrams regarding the case of Irene Rossi list her address as 18 Verraness or Versaness, probably a misspelling of Varennes St., an alley in the Latin Quarter. Running between Union and Green Streets, it is still lined by wood-framed Victorian row houses, nearly identical to and just a block from Jasper Place, where Pietro Spadafora and his mother died.
2. Rupert Blue, Letter to the Surgeon General, February 24, 1904, National Archives and Records Administration, Records Group 90, Central File 1897–1923, Box 617, File 1 of 2.
3. Rupert Blue, Telegram to Wyman, February 17, 1904, NARA, Records Group 90, Central File 1897–1923, Box 617, File 1 of 2.
4. Rupert Blue, Personal Letter to Surgeon General Walter Wyman, February 23, 1904, NARA, Records Group 90, Central File 1897–1923, Box 617, File 1 of 2.
5. Ibid., March 2, 1904, NARA, Records Group 90, Central File 1897–1923, Box 617, File 1 of 2.
6. Ibid., November 30, 1904, NARA, Records Group 90, Central File 1897–1923, Box 617, File 2 of 2.
7. Ibid., July 12, 1904, NARA, Records Group 90, Central File 1897–1923, Box 617, File 1 of 2.
8. Ibid., July 21, 1904, NARA, Records Group 90, Central File 1897–1923, Box 617, File 1 of 2.
9. Ibid., August 18, 1904, NARA, Records Group 90, Central File 1897–1923, Box 617, File 2 of 2.
10. Ibid., January 7, 1905, NARA, Records Group 90, Central File 1897–1923, Box 617, Folder 5608.
11. Resolution of San Francisco Board of Health, February 16, 1905, NARA, Records Group 90, Central File 1897–1923, Box 646, Folder 5608, 1901–1907, Misc., File 2 of 4.
12. Rupert Blue, Letter to Miss Kate Blue, April 26, 1905. Collection of J. Michael Hughes.
13. Ibid., July 18, 1905. Collection of J. Michael Hughes.
14. From William Colby Rucker's unpublished autobiography, "Under the Yellow Flag: Reminiscences of a Sanitarian," p. 8, graciously shared by his grandson Colby Buxton Rucker.

15. Pauline Jacobson, "Specialist Not Blue over the Plague," *San Francisco Bulletin,* February 21, 1908.

16. Rupert Blue, Letter to Kate Lilly Blue, September 3, 1905. Collection of J. Michael Hughes.

17. Rucker, "Under the Yellow Flag," pp. 83–87, courtesy of Colby Buxton Rucker.

18. Rupert Blue, Letter to Miss Kate Blue, September 3, 1905. Collection of J. Michael Hughes.

EARTHQUAKE

1. Gladys Hansen and Emmet Condon, *Denial of Disaster: The Untold Story and Photographs of the San Francisco Earthquake and Fire of 1906* (San Francisco: Cameron and Company, 1989), pp. 13–14. Ms. Hansen, archivist of the city of San Francisco, posted additional quake research on the Web site of the Museum of the City of San Francisco, at www.sfmuseum.org.

2. William Bronson, *The Earth Shook, the Sky Burned* (San Francisco: Chronicle Books, 1986), p. 43.

3. Arnold Genthe, *As I Remember* (New York: A John Day Book, Reynal & Hitchcock, 1936), pp. 88–89.

4. Hansen and Condon, *Denial of Disaster,* p. 49.

5. Malcolm E. Barker, ed., *Three Fearful Days: San Francisco Memoirs of the 1906 Earthquake and Fire* (San Francisco: Londonborn Publications, 1998), p. 137.

6. Hansen and Condon, *Denial of Disaster,* pp. 32–33.

7. Ibid., pp. 73–74.

8. Ibid., p. 43, weighs the reports of atrocities—the real and the apocryphal—as does Bronson, *The Earth Shook, the Sky Burned,* p. 51.

9. George Cooper Pardee, Telegram to Senator George C. Perkins, May 4, 1906, George Cooper Pardee Correspondence and letters, Call Number C-B 400, Box 31, the Bancroft Library, University of California at Berkeley. (Other estimates of losses ranged from $350 million to $1 billion, according to Bronson, *The Earth Shook, the Sky Burned,* p. 108.)

10. Hansen and Condon, *Denial of Disaster,* pp. 152–153. Ms. Hansen's research revised the mortality figures from 498 to about 3,000 dead.

11. Bronson, *The Earth Shook, the Sky Burned,* p. 83.

12. Ibid., pp. 96–116.

13. George Cooper Pardee, Letter to George C. Houghton, Boston, Mass., April 21, 1906, George Cooper Pardee Correspondence and Papers, Call Number C–B400, Box 30, letters written by Pardee from

March 9 to April 21, 1906, Bancroft Library, University of California at Berkeley.

14. Bronson, *The Earth Shook, the Sky Burned,* p. 118.

15. Barker, ed., *Three Fearful Days,* pp. 292–297.

16. Hansen and Condon, *Denial of Disaster,* p. 123.

17. Letter from the army to James W. Ward, president of the Health Commission, May 8, 1906, National Archives and Records Administration, San Bruno, Calif., Records Group 112, Letterman General Hospital, Correspondence and Related Records pertaining to the San Francisco Earthquake and Fire, 1906, Entry 363, Box 1 of 3, Reports (12) of Health Commission, San Francisco.

18. Surgeon General of the Army O'Reilly, Telegram to Torney, Chief Surgeon, Presidio, San Francisco, Calif., April 24 and 25, 1906, NARA, San Bruno, Calif., Records Group 112, Letterman General Hospital, Correspondence and Related Records Pertaining to the San Francisco Earthquake and Fire, 1906, Entry 363, Box 2 of 3, Misc. Correspondence and Directives.

19. Rupert Blue, Letter to Surgeon General Wyman, May 21, 1906, NARA, Records Group 90, Central File 1897–1923, Box 618, File 2 of 3.

"Comfort the People"

1. Walton Bean, *Boss Ruef's San Francisco* (Berkeley: University of California Press, 1952), pp. 152–153.

2. Stranger than fiction, the bizarre denouement of the San Francisco graft trials is too convoluted to detail here. Highlights of the aftermath—including Prosecutor Heney's attempted assassination, Investigator Burns's future as head of the eponymous detective agency, Boss Ruef's and Mayor Schmitz's appeals and abbreviated jail terms, and the latter's amazing return to city politics—are told by Bean, above, pp. 300–316.

3. Minutes of the San Francisco Board of Health, Friday, August 26, 1907, San Francisco Public Library, San Francisco History Center. The incident was also covered in the *San Francisco Call,* August 27, 1907, p. 14, col. 12.

4. F. William Blaisdell, M.D., and Moses Grossman, M.D., *Catastrophes, Epidemics and Neglected Diseases: San Francisco General Hospital and the Evolution of Public Care* (San Francisco: The San Francisco General Hospital Foundation, California Publishing Co., 1999), p. 62.

5. Minutes of the San Francisco Board of Health, September 3, 1907, San Francisco Public Library, San Francisco History Center.

6. Telegram from Mayor Edward Taylor of San Francisco, quoted in President Theodore Roosevelt's Telegram to Surgeon General Wyman, on September 5, 1907, National Archives and Records Administration, Records Group 90, Central File 1897–1923, Box 618, File 1 of 2.

7. Surgeon General Wyman, Telegram to Hon. Edward R. Taylor, Mayor, San Francisco, September 5, 1907, NARA, Records Group 90, Central File 1897–1923, Box 618, File 1 of 2.

8. William Colby Rucker, "Under the Yellow Flag: Reminiscences of a Sanitarian." Unpublished autobiography courtesy of his grandson Colby Buxton Rucker, p. 112.

9. Frank Morton Todd, *Eradicating Plague from San Francisco: A Report of the Citizens' Health Committee and an Account of Its Work* (San Francisco: C. A. Murdock & Co., 1909), p. 38.

10. *Chung Sai Yat Po*, September 12, 1907.

11. Personal communication, Steve Wong, manager of the Hotel St. Francis, photo archives, regarding the hotel's temporary headquarters in quake-shattered Union Square.

12. "No Quarantine Contemplated and No Cause for Alarm Is Found," *San Francisco Call*, September 14, 1907, p. 14, col. 2.

13. Rupert Blue, Letter to the Surgeon General, September 22, 1907, NARA, Records Group 90, Central File 1897–1923, Box 618, File 1 of 2.

14. Blaisdell and Grossman, *Catastrophes, Epidemics and Neglected Diseases*, p. 64.

15. "Examination of Suspected Plague," *Chung Sai Yat Po*, September 13, 1907, p. 2.

The Rattery

1. Rupert Blue, Letter to "Dear Dr. Glennan," September 25, 1907, National Archives and Records Administration, Records Group 90, Central File 1897–1923, Box 618, File 1 of 2.

2. Rupert Blue, "The Underlying Principles of Anti-Plague Measures," *California State Journal of Medicine*, August 1908, reprinted in Frank Morton Todd, *Eradicating Plague from San Francisco: A Report of the Citizens' Health Committee and an Account of Its Works* (San Francisco: C. A. Murdock & Co., 1909), p. 217.

3. Rupert Blue, Circular Letter to San Francisco on rat extermination, October 1, 1907, NARA, Records Group 90, Central File 1897–1923, Box 618, File 1 of 2.

4. Rupert Blue, Telegram to Surgeon General Walter Wyman, October 18, 1907, NARA, Records Group 90, Central File 1897–1923, Box 618, File 1 of 2.

5. Rupert Blue, Letter to Walter Wyman, November 2, 1907, NARA, Records Group 90, Central File 1897–1923, Box 618, File 1 of 2.

6. Rupert Blue, "Rodents in Relation to the Transmission of Bubonic Plague," reprinted in Todd, *Eradicating Plague from San Francisco*, p. 259.

7. Rupert Blue, Letter to the Surgeon General, transmitting necropsy of Margaret Bowers, December 30, 1907, NARA, Records Group 90, Central File 1897–1923, Box 618, File 2 of 2.

8. The tragedy of the Bowers family is told in several contemporary accounts, including a 1908 *Harper's Weekly* article by William Inglis, "The Flea, the Rat and the Plague" which contends that six people died, with only a two-month-old baby surviving. What city and federal records agree upon is that Marguerite and Howard Bowers died of plague, while at least three additional family members sickened and a fourth was hospitalized. For the death toll, this account relies on San Francisco Death Certificates, San Francisco Department of Health, and the autopsy report of Marguerite Bowers sent by Rupert Blue to Walter Wyman on December 30, 1907, on file at the NARA, Records Group 90, Central File 1897–1923, Box 618, File 2 of 2. Documents variously refer to Mrs. Bowers as "Margaret" or "Marguerite."

9. Blue, "The Underlying Principles of Anti-Plague Measures," in Todd, pp. 218–219.

10. "How to Catch Rats," a circular by W. C. Rucker, reprinted in Todd, *Eradicating Plague from San Francisco*, p. 225.

11. Rupert Blue, Letter to Surgeon General Walter Wyman, November 30, 1907, NARA, Records Group 90, Central File 1897–1923, Box 618, File 2 of 2.

12. Rupert Blue, Letter to Mrs. Annie M. Blue, November 19, 1907. Collection of J. Michael Hughes.

13. Rupert Blue, Letter to Surgeon A. H. Glennan, December 2, 1907, NARA, Records Group 90, Central File 1897–1923, Box 618, File 2 of 2.

14. Rupert Blue, Confidential Letter to Dr. Glennan, January 14, 1908, NARA, Records Group 90, Central File 1897–1923, Box 619, File 5608: 1908.

15. "Citizens Urged to War on Rats," *San Francisco Call*, January 29, 1908, p. 7, col. 4.

16. Ibid.

17. William Colby Rucker, "Under the Yellow Flag: Reminiscences of a Sanitarian," unpublished autobiography, courtesy of his grandson Colby Buxton Rucker, p. 118.

18. Todd, *Eradicating Plague from San Francisco*, pp. 85–90 and 296–313.

19. Edna Tartaul Daniel, "Robert Langley Porter: Physician, Teacher and Guardian of the Public Health," University of California Medical Center Library, Archives and Special Collections, Regional Oral History Office, Bancroft Library, University of California, Berkeley, p. 43.

20. Minutes book of the San Francisco Board of Health, February 28, 1908, San Francisco Public Library, History Room.

21. "Orders Slaughter Houses Destroyed," *San Francisco Call*, February 29, 1908.

22. "No Time for Half-Way Measures—CLEAN UP," *San Francisco Examiner*, editorial page, February 14, 1908.

23. Guenter B. Risse, " 'A Long Pull, a Strong Pull, and All Together': San Francisco and Bubonic Plague, 1907–1908," *Bulletin of the History of Medicine* 66 (Spring 1992): 281.

24. "Warn Women Against the Rat Evil," *San Francisco Call*, February 13, 1908, p. 5, col. 1.

25. Rupert Blue, Letter to Kate L. Blue, March 11, 1908. Collection of J. Michael Hughes.

26. "S.P. Men Hunt Rats," *San Francisco Call*, February 19, 1908, p. 7, col. 4.

27. "Thousand a Day Cost of Crusade," *San Francisco Call*, February 15, 1908, p. 4.

28. "Women Continue War on Rats," *San Francisco News*, February 19, 1908, on file in Scrapbook of Citizens' Committee on Plague Eradication, San Francisco Public Library, History Room.

29. Death Certificates of Rachel Voorsanger, January 15, 1908, and Harry Regensburger, January 3, 1908, San Francisco Health Department.

30. Annette Guequierre Rucker, "Woman's Part in the San Francisco Sanitary Crusade." Thanks to Colby Buxton Rucker of Arnold, Md., for sharing his grandmother's essay.

31. "Public Health Up to People," *San Francisco Call*, February 8, 1908, p. 5, col. 3.

32. W. Colby Rucker, "Frisco's Fight with Bubonic Plague," *Technical World Magazine*, 1908, p. 262.

33. Todd, *Eradicating Plague from San Francisco*, pp. 82–83.

34. Rupert Blue, Letter to Mrs. A. M. Blue, February 18, 1908. Collection of J. Michael Hughes.

35. Rucker, "Under the Yellow Flag," p. 122.

36. Daniel, "Robert Langley Porter," p. 50.

37. The rebuilt hospital became the model of public health response to the AIDS epidemic, as discussed in Blaisdell and Grossman, *Catastrophes, Epidemics and Neglected Diseases: San Francisco General Hospital and the Evolution of Public Care* (San Francisco: The San

Francisco General Hospital Foundation, California Publishing Co., 1999).

38. This alfresco fruit feast was recounted in two contemporary accounts in the San Francisco press: " 'Clean-Up' Cheered at Fruit Dinner," *San Francisco Examiner,* March 22, 1908, and "Spread Feast in Sanitary Street," *San Francisco Call,* March 22, 1908.

"Ain't It Awful?"

1. Rupert Blue, Letter to Miss Kate L. Blue, March 11, 1908. Collection of Michael Hughes.
2. Guenter B. Risse, " 'A Long Pull, a Strong Pull, and All Together': San Francisco and Bubonic Plague, 1907–1908," *Bulletin of the History of Medicine* 66 (Spring 1992): 282.
3. Pauline Jacobson, "Specialist Not Blue over the Plague," *San Francisco Bulletin,* February 21, 1908.
4. Ibid.
5. "San Francisco Will Not Be Quarantined," "Great Unit Fighting Filth in Metropolis," and "Laboratory Method of Fighting Plague," a three-part series by Herbert Bashford, *San Jose Mercury,* March 5, 1908, to March 7, 1908.
6. Edna Tartaul Daniel, "Robert Langley Porter: Physician, Teacher and Guardian of the Public Health," University of California Medical Center Library, Archives and Special Collections, Regional Oral History Office, the Bancroft Library, University of California, Berkeley, p. 40. This tart recollection came in an oral-history interview Porter gave Mrs. Daniel at the age of ninety.
7. By the end of the campaign, Blue's cheese purchases alone totaled four thousand pounds a month. Letter to the Surgeon General, December 7, 1908, National Archives and Records Administration, Records Group 90, Central File 1897–1923, Box 619, Folder 5608, File 2 of 3.
8. "Look Out for Colored Rats," *San Francisco Chronicle,* April 8, 1908.
9. Walter Wyman, Personal Letter to P.A. Surgeon Rupert Blue, March 18, 1908, NARA, Records Group 90, Central File 1897–1923, Box 618, File 1 of 3.
10. Coroner's Report of the Death of H. A. Stansfield, April 15, 1908, Office of the Chief Medical Examiner, City and County of San Francisco, Calif. See also "Shoots Himself When Grief Is Unbearable," *San Francisco Chronicle,* April 17, 1908, p. 9, col. 2.
11. "A Mad Scientist," *Wasp* 59, no. 17 (April 25, 1908): 4–5.
12. William Colby Rucker, "Under the Yellow Flag: Reminiscences of a

Sanitarian," unpublished autobiography, courtesy of his grandson Colby Buxton Rucker, p. 113.

13. Ralph Chester Williams, *The United States Public Health Service, 1798–1950* (Washington, D.C.: Commissioned Officers of the United States Public Health Service, 1951), p. 264.

14. C. H. Woolsey, Letter to Rupert Blue, June 24, 1908, National Archives and Records Administration, Records Group 90, Central File 1897–1923, Box 618, File 3 of 3. See also "Rat Inspector Tears Up Flooring for Fun," *San Francisco Chronicle*, April 18, 1908, p. 5, col. 2.

15. Risse, " 'A Long Pull, a Strong Pull, and All Together,' " p. 275.

16. Rupert Blue, Letter to the Surgeon General, April 27, 1908, NARA, Records Group 90, Central File 1897–1923, Box 618, File 3 of 3.

17. Ibid.

18. Gray Brechin, *Imperial San Francisco: Urban Power, Earthly Ruin* (Berkeley: University of California Press, 1999), pp. 162–163.

19. Rupert Blue, Personal Letter to Surgeon General Walter Wyman, May 11, 1908, NARA, Records Group 90, Central File 1897–1923, Box 618, File 2 of 3.

20. Rupert Blue, to Walter Wyman, page 2 of undated fragment, NARA, Records Group 90, Central File 1897–1923, Box 619, Folder 5608: 1908.

21. Rupert Blue, Letter to Walter Wyman, June 19, 1908, NARA, Records Group 90, Central File 1897–1923, Box 618, File 3 of 3.

22. "Bubonic Plague: The Menace of Centuries," *New York Times,* June 14, 1908, sec. 5, p. 2. The victory was prematurely reported in a sidebar headlined TWO LITERARY CLASSICS AND THE PLAGUE.

23. Letter of Rupert Blue to "My Dear Kate," June 26. Collection of J. Michael Hughes. Year not specified, but events discussed and the style of Blue's handwriting sample would place it in 1908.

24. Diary of William Colby Rucker, July 4, 1908, courtesy of Dr. Rucker's grandson Colby Buxton Rucker.

25. Ibid., July 7, 1908.

26. Ibid., July 19, 1908.

27. Mayor Edward Taylor (San Francisco), Letter to Theodore Roosevelt, July 16, 1908, NARA, Records Group 90, Central File 1897–1923, Box 618, File 3 of 3.

28. Colby Rucker Diary, entries of July 27 and 28, 1908.

29. Rupert Blue, Letter to the Surgeon General, August 10, 1908, NARA, Records Group 90, Central File 1897–1923, Box 619, Folder 5608, File 1 of 3.

30. Ibid., August 28, 1908, Records Group 90, Central File 1897–1923, Box 619, File Folder 5608, File 1 of 3.

31. Thanks to Colby Buxton Rucker for sharing his grandfather's typed manuscript of his essay "The Wicked Flea." Additional details on the mating habits of fleas from personal communication, Dr. Kenneth Gage, U.S. Centers for Disease Control and Prevention, Fort Collins, Colo.

32. Charles T. Gregg, *Plague: An Ancient Disease in the Twentieth Century* (Albuquerque: University of New Mexico Press, 1985), pp. 75–77.

33. Carroll Fox, Letter to Rupert Blue, August 26, 1908, NARA, Records Group 90, Central File 1897–1923, Box 619, Folder 5608, File 1 of 3.

34. Rucker Diary, entry of September 16, 1908.

35. Colby Buxton Rucker, personal communication.

36. Rucker Diary, entries of September 17–28, 1908.

37. Frank Morton Todd, *Eradicating Plague from San Francisco: A Report of the Citizens' Health Committee and an Account of Its Works* (San Francisco: C. A. Murdock & Co., 1909), p. 9.

38. Rucker Diary, entry of October 14, 1908.

39. Rucker Diary, entry of October 20, 1908.

THE PIED PIPER

1. *San Francisco Call,* January 5, 1908, as cited in Guenter B. Risse, " 'A Long Pull, a Strong Pull, and All Together': San Francisco and Bubonic Plague, 1907–1908," *Bulletin of the History of Medicine* 66 (Spring 1992): 274.

2. Frank Morton Todd, *Eradicating Plague from San Francisco: A Report of the Citizens' Health Committee and an Account of Its Work* (San Francisco: C. A. Murdock & Co., 1909), p. 9.

3. Ibid., p. 183.

4. "Buffalo Bill in a Moment of Confidence," *Wasp* 60, no. 17 (October 24, 1908): 7.

5. "Clean Bill of Health Given San Francisco: Surgeon General Wyman Reports Pacific States Free from Plague," *San Francisco Call,* November 27, 1908, p. 3, col. 4. (Actually, the headline was misleading, for the city was clean, but plague was migrating east into the countryside.)

6. Rupert Blue, Letter to Kate Lilly Blue, January 20, 1909. Collection of J. Michael Hughes.

7. Details of the fete, covered like a White House dinner, drawn from "Brilliant Banquet in Dr. Blue's Honor," *San Francisco Call,* April 1, 1909, p. 3, col. 1. See also "Homage Paid to Dr. Blue at Big Banquet," *San Francisco Examiner,* April 1, 1909, p. 3, col. 1.

8. Rupert Blue, Letter to General Walter Wyman, February 17, 1909,

National Archives and Records Administration, Records Group 90, Central File 1897–1923, Box 620, Folder 5608, File 1 of 3.

9. William Colby Rucker, "Under the Yellow Flag: Reminiscences of a Sanitarian," unpublished autobiography, courtesy of his grandson Colby Buxton Rucker, p. 130 (inserts numbered 2–5).

10. W. C. Rucker, Letter to Surgeon Rupert Blue, August 12, 1909, NARA, Records Group 90, Central File 1897–1923, Box 626, Folder: Rucker.

11. Rucker, "Under the Yellow Flag," p. 129. Discussing his desperate attempts to guard his son from his wife's tuberculosis by taking him on the road, Rucker wrote: "I thought it better to expose him to this fatigue than to run the chance of picking up his mother's infection. It was a hard summer physically, but mentally it was undiluted anguish. There were periods of [Annette's] improvement followed by greater retrogressions."

12. Rupert Blue, Letter to Surgeon General Wyman, with map of squirrel plague signed "WCR," November 8, 1909, NARA, Records Group 90, Central File 1897–1923, Box 637, Folder: 1899–1909, Surgeon General.

13. Rucker "Under the Yellow Flag," p. 130.

14. Ibid., p. 157. Rucker's tireless campaigning for Blue is also recounted in Bess Furman, *A Profile of the United States Public Health Service, 1798–1948* (Washington, D.C.: U.S. Department of Health, Education, and Welfare, 1973), p. 283. There's a cryptic note in her notebooks, on file at the National Library of Medicine, suggesting that Rucker even lobbied on the golf green with President Taft.

15. "Dr. Blue Assured of Wyman's Job," *San Francisco Call*, January 5, 1912.

16. Rupert Blue, Letter to Miss Kate Blue, December 20, 1911. Collection of J. Michael Hughes.

17. Furman, *A Profile of the United States Public Health Service*, p. 283.

18. Rupert Blue, Letter to the Attorney General, August 27, 1912, Papers of William Howard Taft, Letters, U.S. Library of Congress, Sect. 6(20), Reel 357.

19. Rupert Blue, Letter to Sallie Blue John, December 31, 1912. Collection of J. Michael Hughes.

20. "Health of Public Is Public Utility," *Washington Star*, December 11, 1913, p. 16, col. 1.

21. Ronald L. Numbers, *Almost Persuaded: American Physicians and Compulsory Health Insurance, 1912–1920* (Baltimore: Johns Hopkins University Press, 1978), pp. 52–63.

22. Rupert Blue, Letter to Henriet Blue, August 25, 1914. Collection of J. Michael Hughes.

23. Ralph Chester Williams, *The United States Public Health Service, 1798–1950* (Washington, D.C.: Commissioned Officers Association of the United States Public Health Service, 1951), p. 548.

24. Rupert Blue, Letter to Joseph P. Tumulty, Secretary to the President, February 26, 1919, Papers of Woodrow Wilson, U.S. Library of Congress, Sect. 4, No. 80, Reel 200.

25. Furman, *A Profile of the United States Public Health Service*, pp. 332–335. Furman further suggests that the official charged with appointing Blue's replacement, Treasury Secretary Carter Glass, was himself aspiring to fill a vacant U.S. Senate seat from Virginia and so was influenced in his choice of Cumming, a Virginian, to succeed Blue. Glass subsequently got the Senate appointment.

26. Rupert Blue, Letter to Kate Lilly Blue, June 12, 1923. Collection of J. Michael Hughes.

27. Rucker Diary, March 28, 1924.

28. Colby Buxton Rucker, personal communication.

29. John Stuart Blue, Letter to Kate Lilly Blue, November 6, 1942, Blue Family Papers, South Caroliniana Library, University of South Carolina, Columbia, S.C.

30. Personnel Files of Rupert Blue, on file in Rockville, Md., obtained through assistance of Dr. John Parascandola, historian of the U.S. Public Health Service, and through the filing of a Freedom of Information Act request. See also obituary in *The Washington Post*, "Lillian Latour, 94, Widow of Envoy," June 13, 1977, p. C6. Special thanks to Mary C. Kartman for additional research on Mme. Latour.

31. "Dr. Rupert Blue Laid to Rest," *Marion Star*, editorial page, April 19, 1948.

EPILOGUE

1. John A. Garraty and Mark C. Carnes, *American National Biography*, vol. 12 (New York: Oxford University Press, 1999).

2. Guenter Risse, " 'A Long Pull, a Strong Pull, and All Together': San Francisco and Bubonic Plague, 1907–1908," *Bulletin of the History of Medicine* 66 (Spring 1992): 284–285.

3. Ibid., p. 278. Risse notes that Blue was a "superb politician" with superior PR sense who "spoke softly while brandishing a powerful stick." But when asked in a 2000 interview how Blue, a southerner born and bred, had managed to finesse the racial politics of San Francisco, Elizabeth McIntyre, one of the Marion, South Carolina, senior social observers and a friend of the Blue family, took a different view. "Why," Miss McIntyre replied sweetly, "he had a southern mother."

4. David T. Dennis, Kenneth L. Gage, et al., *Plague Manual: Epidemiol-*

ogy, Distribution, Surveillance and Control (Geneva: World Health Organization, 1999), p. 15. Global case and death reports from 1954 to 1997, and countries with annual plague cases are from the WHO Web site, at www.who.org.

5. Kenneth L. Gage, David T. Dennis, et al., "Cases of Cat-Associated Plague in the Western U.S., 1977–1998," *Clinical Infectious Diseases* 30, no. 6 (June 2000): 893–900.

6. Matt Mygatt, "Woman Contracts Plague After Finding 'Wobbly Mice,' " Associated Press Newswires, January 26, 2000.

7. Kenneth Gage, Centers for Disease Control and Prevention, Fort Collins, Colo., interview with the author, August 24, 2000, by telephone.

8. Interview with bioweapons expert William C. Patrick, former chief of product division, U.S. Army, Fort Detrick, MD, on August 29, 2002.

9. Charles T. Gregg, *Plague: An Ancient Disease in the Twentieth Century* (Albuquerque: University of New Mexico Press, 1985), pp. 211–213. See also R. W. Burmeister et al., "Laboratory-Acquired Pneumonic Plague," *Annals of Internal Medicine* 56, no. 5 (May 1962): 789–800. See also personal communication, Phil Luton, Centre for Applied Microbiology and Research, U.K. Department of Health. Note that the American death occurred while the United States was still actively studying biological weapons, but the British death occurred after the United Kingdom had abandoned its offensive chemical and biological weapons program.

10. Ken Alibek, *Biohazard* (New York: Random House, 1999), pp. 20, 166.

11. J. Parkhill et al., "Genome Sequence of *Yersinia pestis,* the Causative Agent of Plague," *Nature* 413 (October 4, 2001); see also Marilyn Chase, "Researchers in Britain Have Determined the Genetic Sequence of Bubonic Plague," *Wall Street Journal,* October 4, 2001.

12. Rupert Blue, "The Underlying Principles of Anti-Plague Measures," originally published in *California State Journal of Medicine,* 1908, reprinted in Frank Morton Todd, *Eradicating Plague from San Francisco: A Report of the Citizens' Health Committee and an Account of Its Work* (San Francisco: C. A. Murdock & Co., 1909), p. 215.

13. Bess Furman, *A Profile of the United States Public Health Service, 1798–1948* (Washington, D.C.: U.S. Department of Health, Education, and Welfare, 1973), p. 286.

14. Rupert Blue, Letter to Miss Alda Will, August 9, 1912, NARA, Records Group 90, Central File 1897–1923, Box 647, Folder 5608: 1908–12, File 1 of 3.

Bibliography

PRIVATE MANUSCRIPT COLLECTIONS

Letters of Rupert Lee Blue. Collection of J. Michael Hughes, Jacksonville, Fl., great-nephew of Dr. Blue. Quoted by gracious permission of Mr. Hughes.

Blue family letters and memorabilia. Collection of Eleanor Stuart Blue, Washington, D.C., great-niece of Dr. Blue. Quoted by gracious permission of Ms. Blue.

Private papers of W. Colby Rucker. Collection of Colby Buxton Rucker, Arnold, Md., grandson of Dr. Rucker. Quoted by gracious permission of Mr. Rucker.

PUBLIC ARCHIVES

National Archives and Records Administration. Public health documents in Records Group 90, Central File 1897–1923, the NARA II in College Park, Md., and at NARA in San Bruno, Calif.

National Library of Medicine. History of Medicine Division, Bethesda, Md.

The Library of Congress, Washington, D.C.

The Blue Family Collection, including letters of John Gilchrist Blue, Victor Blue, and photographs. The South Caroliniana Library, University of South Carolina, Columbia, S.C.

John Hendricks Kinyoun Papers. Genealogy Series, Rare Book, Manuscript, and Special Collections Library, Duke University, Durham, N.C.

Newspapers

San Francisco Chronicle

San Francisco Examiner

San Francisco Call

The San Francisco News

The Sacramento Bee

San Jose Mercury

The Washington Post

The Washington Star

Chung Sai Yat Po, the daily newspaper of San Francisco Chinatown. Archived on microfilm at the University of California, Berkeley, East Asian Library.

Books

Adams, Charles F. *The Magnificent Rogues of San Francisco: A Gallery of Fakers and Frauds, Rascals and Robber Barons, Scoundrels and Scalawags.* Palo Alto, Calif.: Pacific Books, 1998.

Alibek, Ken. *Biohazard.* New York: Random House, 1999.

Barker, Lewellys F. *Time and the Physician.* New York: G. P. Putnam's Sons, 1942.

Barker, Malcolm E., ed. *San Francisco Memoirs, 1835–1851: Eyewitness Accounts of the Birth of a City.* San Francisco: Londonborn Publications, 1994.

———, ed. *More San Francisco Memoirs, 1852–1899: The Ripening Years.* San Francisco: Londonborn Publications, 1996.

———, ed. *Three Fearful Days: San Francisco Memoirs of the 1906 Earthquake and Fire.* San Francisco: Londonborn Publications, 1998.

Bean, Walton. *Boss Ruef's San Francisco: The Story of the Union Labor Party, Big Business, and the Graft Prosecution.* Berkeley: University of California Press, 1952.

Blaisdell, F. William, M.D., and Moses Grossman, M.D. *Catastrophes, Epidemics and Neglected Diseases: San Francisco General Hospital and the Evolution of Public Care*. San Francisco: The San Francisco General Hospital Foundation, California Publishing Co., 1999.

Boccaccio, Giovanni. *The Decameron*. Trans. Guido Waldman. Oxford: Oxford University Press, 1993.

Brechin, Gray. *Imperial San Francisco: Urban Power, Earthly Ruin*. Berkeley: University of California Press, 1999.

Bronson, William. *The Earth Shook, the Sky Burned: A Photographic Record of the 1906 San Francisco Earthquake and Fire*. San Francisco: Chronicle Books, 1986.

Camus, Albert. *The Plague*. Trans. Stuart Gilbert. New York: Vintage International, 1991.

Cantor, Norman F. *In the Wake of the Plague: The Black Death and the World It Made*. New York: The Free Press, 2001.

Choy, Philip P., Lorraine Dong, and Marlon K. Hom. *The Coming Man: 19th Century Perceptions of the Chinese*. Seattle: University of Washington Press, 1995.

Craddock, Susan. *City of Plagues: Disease, Poverty, and Deviance in San Francisco*. Minneapolis: University of Minnesota Press, 2000.

Defoe, Daniel. *A Journal of the Plague Year*. London: Penguin Books, 1966.

Dennis, David T., Kenneth L. Gage, et al., *Plague Manual: Epidemiology, Distribution, Surveillance and Control*. Geneva: World Health Organization, 1999.

Fracchia, Charles A. *Fire and Gold: The San Francisco Story*. Encinitas, Calif.: Heritage Media Corp., 1996.

Furman, Bess. *A Profile of the United States Public Health Service, 1798–1948*. Washington, D.C.: U.S. Department of Health, Education, and Welfare, 1973.

Garraty, John A., and Mark C. Carnes. *American National Biography*. New York: Oxford University Press, 1999.

Genthe, Arnold. *As I Remember*. New York: A John Day Book, Reynal & Hitchcock, 1936.

Gregg, Charles T. *Plague: An Ancient Disease in the Twentieth Century*. Albuquerque: University of New Mexico Press, 1985.

Hammond, Peter M., and Gradon B. Carter. *From Biological Warfare to Healthcare: Porton Down, 1940–2000*. Hampshire, England: Palgrave, 2002.

Hansen, Gladys, and Emmet Condon. *Denial of Disaster: The Untold Story and Photographs of the San Francisco Earthquake and Fire of 1906.* San Francisco: Cameron and Company, 1989.

Harden, Victoria A. *Inventing the NIH: Federal Biomedical Research Policy, 1887–1937.* Baltimore: Johns Hopkins University Press, 1986.

Hart, James D. *A Companion to California.* New York: Oxford University Press, 1978.

Hodgson, Barbara. *The Rat: A Perverse Miscellany.* Berkeley: Ten Speed Press, 1997.

Hom, Marlon K. *Songs of Gold Mountain: Cantonese Rhymes from San Francisco Chinatown.* Berkeley: University of California Press, 1987.

Lai, Him Mark, Genny Lim, and Judy Yung. *Island: Poetry and History of Chinese Immigrants on Angel Island, 1910–1940.* Seattle: University of Washington Press, 1991.

Lau, Theodora. *The Handbook of Chinese Horoscopes.* New York: Perennial Library, 1988.

Levy, Harriet Lane. *920 O'Farrell Street: A Jewish Girlhood in Old San Francisco.* Berkeley: Heyday Books, 1996.

Lewis, Sinclair. *Arrowsmith.* New York: Signet Classic, 1961.

Martin, Mildred Crowl. *Chinatown's Angry Angel: The Story of Donaldina Cameron.* Palo Alto, Calif.: Pacific Books, 1986.

Mayne, Alan. *The Imagined Slum: Newspaper Representation in Three Cities, 1870–1914.* Leicester: Leicester University Press, 1993.

McClain, Charles J. *In Search of Equality: The Chinese Struggle Against Discrimination in Nineteenth-Century America.* Berkeley: University of California Press, 1994.

McNeill, William H. *Plagues and Peoples.* New York: Anchor Books/ Doubleday, 1977.

Melendy, H. Brett, and Benjamin F. Gilbert. *The Governors of California: Peter H. Burnett to Edmund G. Brown.* Georgetown, Calif.: The Talisman Press, 1965.

The Merck Manual. 17th ed. Edited by Mark H. Beers, M.D., and Robert Berkow, M.D. Whitehouse Station, N.J.: Merck Research Laboratories, 1999.

Merck's 1899 Manual. New York: Merck & Co., 1899.

Mollaret, Henri H., and Jacqueline Brossolet. *Alexandre Yersin, ou Le vainqueur de la peste.* Paris: Librairie Artheme Fayard, 1985.

Mullan, Fitzhugh. *Plagues and Politics: The Story of the United States Public Health Service.* New York: Basic Books, 1989.

Nee, Victor G., and Brett de Bary Nee. *Longtime Californ': A Documentary Study of an American Chinatown.* Stanford: Stanford University Press, 1986.

Numbers, Ronald L. *Almost Persuaded: American Physicians and Compulsory Health Insurance, 1912–1920.* Baltimore: Johns Hopkins University Press, 1978.

O'Brien, Robert. *This Is San Francisco.* San Francisco: Chronicle Books, 1994.

Pierce, J. Kingston. *San Francisco, You're History!* Seattle: Sasquatch Books, 1995.

Porter, Roy. *The Greatest Benefit to Mankind: A Medical History of Humanity.* New York: W. W. Norton & Co., 1997.

Rathmell, George. *Realms of Gold: The Colorful Writers of San Francisco, 1850–1950.* Berkeley: Creative Arts Book Company, 1998.

Rucker, W. Colby. "Under the Yellow Flag: Reminiscences of a Sanitarian." This unpublished autobiography of Dr. Rucker's was graciously shared by his grandson Colby Buxton Rucker of Arnold, Md.

Tchen, John Kuo Wei. *Genthe's Photographs of San Francisco's Old Chinatown.* Photographs by Arnold Genthe. New York: Dover Publications, 1984.

Todd, Frank Morton. *Eradicating Plague from San Francisco: A Report of the Citizens' Health Committee and an Account of Its Work.* San Francisco: C. A. Murdock & Co., 1909.

Twain, Mark. *The Innocents Abroad.* New York: Signet Classic, 1966.

———. *The Complete Humorous Sketches and Tales of Mark Twain.* Edited by Charles Neider. Cambridge, Mass.: Da Capo Press, 1996.

Williams, Ralph Chester. *The United States Public Health Service, 1798–1950.* Washington, D.C.: Commissioned Officers Association of the United States Public Health Service, 1951.

Yung, Judy. *Unbound Feet: A Social History of Chinese Women in San Francisco.* Berkeley: University of California Press, 1995.

——. *Unbound Voices: A Documentary History of Chinese Women in San Francisco.* Berkeley: University of California Press, 1999.

Ziegler, Philip. *The Black Death.* Surrey, Eng.: Sutton Publishing Ltd., Bramley Books, Quadrillion Publishing Ltd., 1998.

ARTICLES, MONOGRAPHS, ORAL HISTORIES

Daniel, Edna Tartaul. "Robert Langley Porter: Physician, Teacher and Guardian of the Public Health." University of California, San Francisco, Medical Center Library, Archives and Special Collections. Permission to quote granted by Regional Oral History Office, Bancroft Library, University of California, Berkeley.

Link, Vernon B. "A History of Plague in the United States." Public Health Monograph no. 26. Washington, D.C.: U.S. Public Health Service, 1955.

Lipson, George Loren. "Plague in San Francisco in 1900: The United States Marine Hospital Service Commission to Study the Existence of Plague in San Francisco." *Annals of Internal Medicine* 77, no. 2 (August 1972): 303–310.

Lucaccini, Luigi F. "The Public Health Service on Angel Island." *Public Health Reports* 3 (January/February 1996): 92–94.

"The Report of the Government Commission on the Existence of Plague in San Francisco." *Occidental Medical Times* XV, no. 4 (April 1901): 101–117.

Risse, Guenter B. " 'A Long Pull, a Strong Pull, and All Together': San Francisco and Bubonic Plague, 1907–1908." *Bulletin of the History of Medicine* 66 (Spring 1992): 260–286.

——. "The Politics of Fear: Bubonic Plague in San Francisco, California, 1900." In *New Countries and Old Medicine: Proceedings of an International Conference on the History of Medicine and Health,* edited by Linda Bryder and Derek A. Dow, pp. 1–19. Auckland, New Zealand: Pyramid Press, 1995.

Scholten, Paul. "When Bubonic Plague Came to San Francisco." *San Francisco Medicine* (July 1980), 16–18.

Trauner, Joan B. "The Chinese as Medical Scapegoats in San Francisco, 1870–1905." *California History* 57, no. 1 (Spring 1978): 70–87.

Wyman, Walter. *The Bubonic Plague.* Washington, D.C.: Government Printing Office, 1900.

Index

A Note on the Type

This book was set in Fairfield, the first typeface from the hand of the distinguished American artist and engraver Rudolph Ruzicka (1883–1978). In its structure, Fairfield displays the sober and sane qualities of the master craftsman whose talent has long been dedicated to clarity. It is this trait that accounts for the trim grace and vigor, the spirited design, and sensitive balance of this original typeface.

Rudolph Ruzicka was born in Bohemia and came to America in 1894. He set up his own shop, devoted to wood engraving and printing, in New York in 1913, after a varied career working as a wood engraver, in photo-engraving and banknote-printing plants, and as an art director and freelance artist. He designed and illustrated many books, and was the creator of a considerable list of individual prints—wood engravings, line engravings on copper, and aquatints.